COVID-19

by Edward K. Chapnick, MD

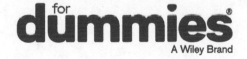

for
dummies®
A Wiley Brand

COVID-19 For Dummies®

Published by: **John Wiley & Sons, Inc.**, 111 River Street, Hoboken, NJ 07030-5774, www.wiley.com

Copyright © 2024 by John Wiley & Sons, Inc., Hoboken, New Jersey

Media and software compilation copyright © 2024 by John Wiley & Sons, Inc. All rights reserved.

Published simultaneously in Canada

For general information on our other products and services, please contact our Customer Care Department within the U.S. at 877-762-2974, outside the U.S. at 317-572-3993, or fax 317-572-4002. For technical support, please visit https://hub.wiley.com/community/support/dummies.

Wiley publishes in a variety of print and electronic formats and by print-on-demand. Some material included with standard print versions of this book may not be included in e-books or in print-on-demand. If this book refers to media such as a CD or DVD that is not included in the version you purchased, you may download this material at http://booksupport.wiley.com. For more information about Wiley products, visit www.wiley.com.

Library of Congress Control Number: 2023947192

ISBN 978-1-394-21171-5 (pbk); ISBN 978-1-394-21172-2 (ePub); ISBN 978-1-394-21173-9 (ePDF)

SKY10057407_101223

Contents at a Glance

Table of Contents

Introduction

COVID-19 For Dummies is here to give you all of the vital information about COVID-19 without conflicting opinions or complex biology lessons. In this book, you can get everything you need to know about COVID-19 in one place — from the way the virus works and details on the pandemic of 2020, to how to protect yourself and others from the disease. And you can even discover insights about what experts think the future holds for COVID-19.

About This Book

What sets this book apart from other books on this subject is that it truly combines history of the 2020 pandemic, the science of viruses, public health and safety, and my own personal stories and thoughts as an Infectious Diseases Specialist. I've been on the frontlines of many epidemics, and I was there (and still am) during and after the COVID-19 pandemic swept the world. I take you behind the scenes of the medical world to share lessons, tips, and ideas for how to continue to co-exist with COVID-19 in a healthy way.

I organize this book in the same way that all For Dummies books are organized. That means it includes straightforward and functional chapter titles and headings that tell you exactly what information each chapter and section covers, many bulleted lists and numbered steps to make the information easy to find and digest, and a friendly tone free of lingo and medical jargon.

I also use special formatting conventions to call out certain content:

>> Web addresses appear in monofont. If you're reading a digital version of this book on a device connected to the Internet, note that you can click the web address to visit that website, like this: www.dummies.com.

>> Italicized text means that you are reading a new term or definition.

>> Words in **bold** highlight a step in a process.

To make the content more accessible, I divided this book into four parts:

>> **Part 1: Understanding COVID-19 Basics.** This part includes chapters that give you all of the information about how the virus works, as well as historical details about what happened during the 2020 pandemic.

>> **Part 2: Staying Safe and Healthy.** This part tells you how to prevent the spread of COVID-19 and what to do if you experience symptoms. And in this part, you can also find a chapter dedicated solely to what Long COVID is and how to deal with it.

>> **Part 3: Accepting COVID-19 Is Here to Stay.** This part details what the world looks like after the 2020 pandemic. Chapters in this part address what to expect going forward in a world that contains COVID-19, as well as how to stay safe at work and in other public places.

>> **Part 4: The Part of Tens.** The Part of Tens is a *For Dummies* special. This part gives you several chapters that provide bonus lists of (usually) ten tips, tricks, secrets, or other thoughts that you can to use to further your knowledge of COVID-19 and contribute to the betterment of public health overall.

Foolish Assumptions

I try not to make assumptions in life, but admittedly, I've written this book assuming that you know at least that COVID-19 exists and that you probably lived through the 2020 pandemic. Here are some other possible assumptions:

>> COVID-19 is somehow currently impacting you personally, or has impacted you in the past — otherwise, you probably wouldn't be here.

>> You respect and trust science and medical evidence. (This book is firmly rooted in both.)

>> You're probably not a medical professional, but rather, a world citizen looking for a quick and easy read of complex subject matter.

I keep the information and presentation as simple as possible. I leave out any advanced scientific and medical coverage that's beyond the scope of the book. After all, this isn't a medical school textbook!

Icons Used in This Book

Throughout this book, icons in the margins highlight certain types of valuable information that call out for your attention. Here are the icons you encounter and a brief description of each.

TIP

The Tip icon marks my practical ideas and actions that you can take on all things related to COVID-19. They could be prevention tips, ways to take care of yourself if you're sick with COVID-19, or tricks for staying up to date on the latest COVID-19 news.

REMEMBER

Remember icons mark the information that's especially important to know. To grab the most important information in each chapter at a glance, just skim through the paragraphs marked with these icons.

WARNING

The Warning icon tells you to watch out and pay close attention. It marks important information that's often related to health or medical safety issues. Always read this information!

Beyond the Book

In addition to the abundance of information and guidance related to COVID-19 that I provide in this book, you get access to even more help and information online at Dummies.com. Check out this book's online Cheat Sheet. Just go to www.dummies.com and search for "COVID-19 For Dummies Cheat Sheet."

Where to Go from Here

Like all *For Dummies* books, this book isn't linear — you can start anywhere and read the chapters in any order that you want. You can even skip some! You don't need to read all of the early chapters in order to understand the later ones. If you might benefit from information that I discuss elsewhere in the book, I do my best to give you a quick refresher or a cross-reference to another chapter that holds additional information.

If you're reading this book, I know it's possible that you or someone you know has COVID-19, and you need the right info right away, so let me offer you this quick-start guide. Turn to

>> Chapter 7 if you tested positive for COVID-19 and need to know what to do next

>> Chapter 8 if you have symptoms of COVID-19 and need to know whether you should seek treatment

>> Chapter 5 if you want to know whether your symptoms indicate a cold, the flu, or COVID-19

>> Chapter 9 if you've already had COVID-19 and recovered, but you're still experiencing symptoms weeks, months, or even years later

And, of course, you can always check out the Table of Contents and the Index to find the coverage you're specifically looking for.

1

Understanding COVID-19 Basics

Survey COVID-19 on a personal and global level.

Discover how the SARS-CoV-2 and other viruses in the coronavirus family function.

Get a sense of what happened during the height of the 2020 pandemic.

Look at how countries around the world are currently managing COVID-19.

Chapter **1**
COVID-19 in a Nutshell

n the winter of 2019, an unknown virus started making people sick in Wuhan, China. Within weeks, scientists identified the virus as SARS-CoV-2 and saw it spread beyond Wuhan. The viral infection quickly snowballed into one of the most transformative global events of the 21st century: the 2020 COVID-19 pandemic.

The pandemic wasn't just a health problem; it penetrated every facet of societies across the world. The pandemic revealed vulnerabilities in healthcare systems, stoked public fears and mistrust of ever-changing public health policies, and caused millions of deaths worldwide. At the same time, people rose up to meet the challenges. Communities came together to support one another emotionally and logistically. Healthcare and essential workers kept medical facilities, stores, and other infrastructure operating, despite enormous obstacles.

As an Infectious Diseases specialist since 1991, I worked through the HIV, H1N1, SARS, smallpox, and Ebola epidemics, and I was also on the frontlines for COVID-19. In this book, I cover the basics of COVID-19, from its insidious beginnings to its widespread ramifications. I also give you my own personal insight and experience as a medical worker during this pandemic.

Going Over the Basics

The amount of information to know about COVID-19 can feel overwhelming because you can find just so much of it out there — plus, some of it changes from time to time, while scientists discover more about the disease.

In this section, I give you a quick glance at the foundation of COVID-19, from the basic science of the virus, to how people transmit it, to uncovering why this virus remains a concern for people worldwide.

MY PERSONAL THOUGHTS ON THE PANDEMIC: WHY SO MUCH ANGER?

The 2020 pandemic was unique, and my personal experience during its run was quite different from my experience during previous epidemics (the Ebola epidemic of 2014, for example). In addition to the normal fear and stress that many healthcare workers (and the general public) felt, I also found that I felt (and sometimes still feel) immense anger, which was a unique emotion for me related to the practice of medicine.

This anger comes from knowing that the 2020 COVID-19 pandemic didn't have to happen — or, at the very least, didn't have to happen with the severity it did. I can't understand or condone how some of numerous individuals and institutions put in place to protect the world's population against widespread infection ended up utterly failing humanity in 2020 and 2021.

Now, I wish to emphasize that many members of various health, government, and other public institutions and entities went above and beyond the call of duty during this time. However, from my viewpoint, a significant enough minority of people across these entities gave in to fear, ignorance, personal gain, incompetence, political advancement, and pure arrogance. As a result, the world had to face a pandemic that was much worse than it had to be.

I write this book through that lens, and I present a mix of history and science of the virus itself, as well as a retelling and analysis of how the pandemic reshaped people's perceptions of community, economy, politics, and self.

Recognizing COVID-19 and global responses

COVID-19 is a highly contagious respiratory illness caused by a coronavirus (a large family of respiratory viruses) called SARS-CoV-2. Here's what the name COVID-19 means:

>> **COVI:** Coronavirus

>> **D:** Disease

>> **19:** 2019 (the year it was discovered)

A lot of evidence suggests that the virus started in animals in Wuhan, China, and jumped to humans in late 2019. (If you want to read more about how scientists think that jump happened, turn to Chapter 3.) Although doctors now have several ways to treat the virus, new variants of COVID-19 continue to emerge, making COVID-19 an ever-present global health concern.

REMEMBER

COVID-19 affects each person differently. Some individuals experience mild symptoms, such as fever, cough, and fatigue, while others experience more severe manifestations, such as pneumonia, respiratory failure, and in some cases, even death.

Because of the severity of symptoms and the death toll resulting from the 2020 COVID-19 pandemic, most countries' governments (at country-wide and local levels) enacted public health policies and practices to contain its spread, including

>> **Widespread testing,** which was often available free of charge during the height of the pandemic

>> **Isolation measures** for people who had the disease

>> **Quarantine measures** for people exposed to the virus

>> **Public safety practices,** such as social-distancing and wearing masks

Also, governments and agencies supported the rapid development of vaccines to offer protection against COVID-19.

To read more on the global impact of the pandemic, turn to Chapter 4.

Understanding who's most vulnerable

Adults over the age of 65 and individuals who have underlying health conditions have a higher risk for contracting and experiencing severe illness or complications from COVID-19. Common *comorbidities* (conditions or diseases that occur simultaneously with another) that make people more vulnerable to the virus include

>> Chronic respiratory diseases

>> Compromised immune systems

>> Diabetes

>> Heart disease

>> Obesity

Additionally, factors such as poverty, inadequate access to healthcare or nutrition, crowded living situations, and language and cultural barriers can also heighten people's susceptibility to becoming ill with COVID-19.

Grasping the global concern

You'd be hard pressed to find a corner of the globe that COVID-19 hasn't touched. Maybe some remote villages and isolated tribes have remained unscathed, but for the majority of cities, towns, and villages around the world, COVID-19 became a huge health crisis during 2020 and 2021.

As of this writing, governments, public health agencies, doctors, and scientists have gotten the virus under control enough that the World Health Organization (WHO) no longer considers it a *pandemic* (meaning it's an illness spread across many regions around the world at the same time, disrupting public health, the economy, and daily life). Still, you can expect COVID-19 to remain a part of life because

>> People can easily spread the SARS-CoV-2 virus to each other through coughs, sneezes, or even just talking in close proximity.

>> International travel allows people from all countries to potentially spread viruses, turning isolated outbreaks into widespread contagion within weeks.

>> The SARS-CoV-2 virus has the potential to cause severe illness and hospitalizations for some people — and if not managed well, may overwhelm healthcare systems and cause a high number of fatalities again.

>> Scientists continue to study and find out more about the original virus, and all of the variants that continue to emerge. Future variants may not be responsive to vaccines and prevention.

The truth is, the world will most likely see another pandemic, even if it's not COVID-19. To discover some of my ideas and suggestions for how countries around the world can prevent and prepare for the next pandemic, visit Chapter 14.

Knowing how COVID-19 spreads

People infected with COVID-19 primarily transmit it to others through aerosol or respiratory droplets that they emit when they cough, sneeze, talk, or breathe on someone else. If you're infected and in close physical contact with another person, that person may inhale droplets that you exhale.

Additionally, people can contract the virus by having an infected droplet land on their hands and then touching their face, particularly their eyes, nose, or mouth.

Turn to Chapter 5 if you want further detail about how people transmit COVID-19, including information about the difference between aerosol and droplet transmission, how surfaces aren't the danger that we in the medical community once thought they were, and the characteristics of superspreader events.

Coping with COVID-19

COVID-19 isn't going anywhere. As of this writing, most people can look at COVID-19 as a minor health concern, but that doesn't mean people should become complacent. Stay up to date on the latest about symptoms, prevention, and treatment to ensure that the world doesn't see a repeat of a pandemic like the one in 2020.

In the following sections, I give you information about the basic symptoms to watch for, as well as recommendations on minimizing the spread of COVID-19, getting tested if you think you do have it, seeking treatment, and managing Long COVID if you have to.

Surveying the symptoms

The trickiest part of diagnosing (and treating) COVID-19 may be that its symptoms vary so widely in severity and duration — and they're often similar to or the same as other illnesses, such as a cold or the flu. Everyone experiences the onset and progression of symptoms, typically appearing 2 to 14 days after exposure, differently; so if you want to lessen your chance of getting severely ill, you must monitor yourself for symptoms and detect COVID-19 as early as possible.

REMEMBER

Although many individuals experience mild symptoms, some people can develop severe respiratory and systemic complications. Some common mild symptoms that you may feel if you have COVID-19 are

>> Congestion

>> Cough

>> Diarrhea

>> Fatigue

>> Fever or chills

>> Headache

>> Muscle or body aches

WARNING

Some symptoms of COVID-19 are severe enough that they may require you to go a hospital or other medical facility immediately, and include

>> Bluish lips or face

>> Confusion or inability to stay awake

>> Difficulty breathing or shortness of breath

>> Persistent chest pain or pressure

>> Persistent dizziness or lightheadedness

Keep in mind, the preceding lists give you only a quick overview. You may find the symptoms and impacts of COVID-19 confusing and sometimes very concerning. To read more about symptoms in detail — including how they compare to symptoms of a cold and the flu — turn to Chapter 5.

Keeping yourself and others safe

Even though COVID-19 is no longer considered a pandemic by the WHO as of this writing, and public health agencies and public businesses have relaxed their masking and social distance policies, you still have many ways that you can prevent spreading or contracting COVID-19. For example, you can

>> **Wear a mask,** especially indoors or in crowded spaces where maintaining adequate social distancing poses a challenge. Masks significantly decrease the chance that you'll exhale potentially infectious respiratory droplets onto someone else — or inhale their infectious droplets.

>> **Wash your hands regularly** with soap and water for at least 20 seconds — or use hand sanitizers containing at least 60 percent alcohol — to eliminate risks associated with touching contaminated objects.

>> **Improve ventilation** at work, home, or other indoor areas to disperse any viral particles more effectively. The more the air moves, the more germs move away from you.

>> **Get vaccinated.** Vaccines can prevent severe illness, transmission of the virus, and hospitalization.

>> **Stay updated on local COVID-19 trends and guidelines,** and adjust your behaviors based on the best available public health recommendations.

For more ideas, tips, and tricks about preventing yourself and others from spreading COVID-19, visit Chapter 6.

Getting tested

If you're feeling under the weather, were close to someone who tested positive for COVID-19, or recently attended a crowded event, get tested for the virus. And if you plan to travel or join a big gathering, you can always take a test to make sure that you aren't going to spread the virus without knowing it.

As of this writing, various tests are available, and each has pros and cons to using them. The COVID-19 tests also have unique ideal times for taking them to achieve the most accurate results. For more information about how each type of test works — and how to choose and use them — visit Chapter 7.

To get tested, you may be able to visit your local health department, community clinics, pharmacies, or your doctor's office. Many locations offer walk-in appointments, but scheduling your test ahead of time can save you time. Some places even provide drive-through testing, so you don't even have to leave your car.

TIP

If you prefer using a home test, numerous online platforms ship testing kits right to your doorstep. Some test kits give you rapid results within 15 minutes, while others require that you send your sample to a lab by using the provided kit. No matter which method you choose, make sure that you follow the test instructions closely.

Seeking treatment

I cover treatment for COVID-19 in detail in Chapter 8, but here, I'd like to say that getting the right treatment for COVID-19 can make all the difference in your recovery journey. If you have

>> **Mild symptoms:** If you've tested positive and have only mild symptoms, you probably can manage your illness at home by isolating, getting plenty of rest, staying hydrated, taking over-the-counter medication, and monitoring your symptoms.

>> **Severe symptoms or underlying health conditions:** You may need to see your doctor for treatment, which may include hospitalization.

REMEMBER

The good news is that we in the medical community continue to refine our treatments and therapies while we discover more about the virus. If you suspect you have COVID-19 or are experiencing worsening symptoms, don't hesitate to contact a healthcare provider for guidance and potential treatment options.

Managing Long COVID

One of the characteristics that sets COVID-19 apart from many other viruses is the length of time that symptoms can last for some people. Even after recovering from your initial illness, you may experience lingering or new symptoms for months — or even years. Living with Long COVID can feel like running a marathon, but remember, you're not alone on this journey. Many people are navigating the challenges of Long COVID, and like them, you can find strength in community and adaptive routines.

Although you may find managing Long COVID daunting, you can find a wealth of resources and professionals eager to help. Regularly check in with your healthcare provider to discuss symptoms and get advice on managing them. Your provider might recommend physical therapy, counseling, or other supportive treatments to help you regain strength and overall well-being.

TIP

If you have Long COVID, remember that every day is a new day. Embrace the support from loved ones and the community at large, and believe in your resilience and capacity to adapt. You've got this!

If you or someone you know is living with Long COVID and would like more guidance, turn to Chapter 9.

Recovering from COVID-19

Bouncing back from COVID-19 is a unique journey for everyone, so while you get back on your feet, you have to listen to your body. If you feel tired, take that well-deserved nap. Hungry for some fresh air? Consider short, gentle walks outdoors. Keeping a positive mindset, staying hydrated, and eating nutritious foods can help boost your recovery speed. And if you ever feel overwhelmed, remember to reach out to friends, family, or support groups — they're cheering for you, and they want to help!

REMEMBER

Your post-COVID journey might come with its ups and downs, but every day is progress. Help your progress along by

>> **Staying in touch with your healthcare provider:** They can offer guidance tailored to your recovery and answer any lingering questions. Your healthcare provider is your trusted partner in this process.

>> **Reintroducing daily routines:** Getting back into your normal routine is a great idea, but don't rush it — take things at your own pace. Before you know it, you're back to your vibrant self, with a newfound appreciation for health and the small joys of life.

Here are some clues that you may be on the other side of COVID-19. You have

>> No more shortness of breath or difficulty in breathing.

>> No fever for at least 24 hours without the use of fever-reducing medications.

>> Improved energy levels and less fatigue.

>> No more confusion, as well as having improved concentration and what you feel is a normal mental state.

>> Reduced or eliminated cough or body aches.

TIP

Before returning to work or interacting with others, make sure you read Chapter 7, where I dive deep into the timelines of testing, waiting until you're symptom-free (or at least your symptoms are improving), and ensuring that you keep others safe during your return.

If you find yourself with a sticky work situation, such as your supervisor pressuring you to return to work when you are not healthy, and need guidance about your federal rights under the Americans with Disabilities Act as it pertains to COVID-19, see Chapter 9.

Considering the Future of COVID-19

Nobody can truly predict the future, of course, but as of this writing, many of us epidemiologists and other health experts have various hopes, expectations, and beliefs regarding a future that includes COVID-19.

Hopes

Health experts are hopeful that SARS-CoV-2, the virus causing COVID-19, will eventually become *endemic*, as declared by WHO. This means that it could circulate within human populations for years but might become a more regular, predictable, and potentially less severe disease over time, similar to the seasonal flu.

One silver lining of the pandemic continues to serve public health well. Many people have adopted behaviors such as frequent handwashing, mask-wearing in crowded places or during illness, and working remotely. All of these practices can help keep germs at bay.

Expectations

Medical providers expect that vaccines will continue to play a crucial role in protecting the world's population from COVID-19, similar to annual flu shots. Booster shots will most likely remain a recommended practice because the world will probably have to always deal with new variants while they emerge naturally over time.

The development of the COVID-19 vaccine is also a silver lining. Never before have people in the medical field been able to develop a vaccine for a new illness so quickly. The technology used for the COVID-19 vaccine enables the medical community to make new vaccines much more quickly, including better vaccines for childhood illnesses and perhaps even for some types of cancer. For more on how the pandemic sparked innovations in vaccine and other technologies, flip to Chapter 13.

Beliefs

Medical researchers believe that the key to keeping ahead of COVID-19 involves seeing whether variants are more transmissible or cause more severe disease. As long as governments and public health agencies continue their ongoing surveillance and genetic sequencing, the world can continue to detect and understand these variants, providing new vaccines, early warnings, and current medical data to the global community.

Even though COVID-19 is much more controlled now (as of this writing) than it was in 2020, we in the medical community believe that sporadic outbreaks can happen, especially in pockets of unvaccinated individuals or areas that have limited access to vaccines. The scale and severity of these outbreaks depends on various factors, including the level of population immunity and the nature of circulating variants.

SALUTING THE PANDEMIC HEROES

Despite my description in the sidebar "My personal thoughts on the pandemic: Why so much anger?" in this chapter — where I discuss that governments and organizations didn't do many things correctly during the 2020 COVID-19 pandemic — I'm incredibly proud of the healthcare workers, first responders, workers in retail and food service, and all of those who couldn't work from home and who still came to work every day. These people are the true heroes of the pandemic and are the only reason most of us made it through the pandemic at all.

Moving forward

I've gathered many lessons that the medical community learned from the COVID-19 pandemic, and I offer suggestions for how the global community can prevent and prepare for the next pandemic. Flip to Chapter 14 to find out more.

And visit Chapter 13 if you want to read more about the ways in which COVID-19 has changed the world. Some of them may be part of your own life now, and others may come as a total surprise.

REMEMBER

COVID-19 remains dynamic, with ongoing research refining our understanding of the virus and its implications. Keep informed through reliable and authoritative sources while the world, the virus, and our understanding of both evolve. So, stay tuned to announcements from sources such as the Centers for Disease Control and Prevention (CDC), your local health department, and the World Health Organization (WHO).

Chapter **2**

Uncovering the Science of COVID-19

R emember when the word COVID meant nothing to the average person? In today's world — where COVID is ubiquitous across the globe — our pre-pandemic days can seem like a lifetime ago.

The Coronavirus Disease of 2019 (COVID-19) devastated populations around the world when it first arrived *because we knew so little about it.* Now that we know more, we can empower ourselves with the facts. Knowing all that we can about this illness and its virus makes us all stronger. And even though COVID is now a large part of our lives, while researchers make new discoveries, doctors try new treatments, and patients experience different symptoms, keeping up with how the virus works can be challenging.

In this chapter, I try to help you overcome that challenge. I lay out the basic science of the virus that causes COVID-19, introduce you to the coronavirus family, and go over the key reasons why COVID-19 is different from the other viruses in its family.

Getting to Know the Coronavirus Family

COVID-19 is an illness caused by a virus called Severe Acute Respiratory Syndrome Coronavirus 2 (SARS-CoV-2). This virus is part of the coronavirus family.

This family includes seven types of coronaviruses that cause intestinal and respiratory illness in people and several more that affect just animals. Some coronaviruses, known as *zoonotic* viruses, can transfer from animals to people. Zoonotic viruses tend to be more dangerous than species-specific viruses because our immune system has not seen them or anything like them, so we do not have immunity against them.

Often, the trouble starts when many different species of animals live within close proximity to each other, and then get sick. If one species has a virus, it can recombine with a different virus from a different species, essentially making a whole new virus that is extra contagious and virulent since it is new to all species. And if humans come into contact with animals that have these new combinations of viruses, they can potentially contract them, and then pass them on to other humans.

We don't know for sure, but scientists suspect that many human viruses, including influenza, human immunodeficiency viruses (HIV), and Monkeypox virus (Mpox), began this way. And yep — you guessed it — SARS (and therefore, COVID-19) is most likely zoonotic. The other well-known zoonotic coronavirus is Middle East Respiratory Syndrome (MERS).

Examining coronavirus structure

To understand how coronaviruses work, start by looking at their physical structure. As shown in Figure 2-1, coronaviruses are spherical in shape and have little bits of protein that protrude from the sphere in all directions. The protrusions, which are also known as *spike proteins,* make it extra easy for the virus to penetrate, bind to, and infect healthy cells. This property is one of the biggest reasons coronaviruses are so contagious.

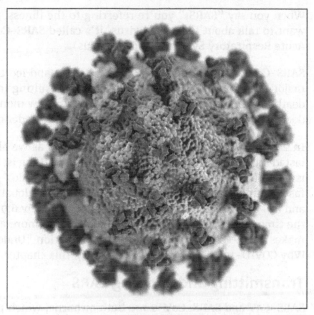

CDC/Alissa Eckert, MSMI; Dan Higgins, MAMS; 2020

FIGURE 2-1: The spikes of protein on the spherical body of the coronavirus makes it both very contagious and easy for your immune system to detect.

But at the same time, those spike proteins can be a good thing because they help your immune system detect the virus easily and mount a defense right away. Also, scientists have found that they can use these spike proteins to create vaccines for COVID-19 (more on that in the section "Surveying the Science of Vaccines," later in this chapter).

Coronaviruses are also *enveloped*, which means they wrap themselves in a membrane they make by taking a part of the host cell's membrane when they reproduce. These membranes make the coronavirus stick to surfaces, so they're susceptible to elimination by disinfectants.

Sizing up SARS

Severe Acute Respiratory Syndrome (SARS) is both the virus and the illness. The distinction between the two is in the terminology.

When you say "SARS," you're referring to the illness, and if you want to talk about the actual virus, it's called SARS-CoV (Severe Acute Respiratory Syndrome Coronavirus).

SARS-CoV originally began in China in 2003 and led to the first major illness outbreak of the 21st century, resulting in over 700 deaths. Thankfully, the outbreak lasted only a few months before doctors, health officials, and citizens brought it under control.

REMEMBER

In 2019, SARS-CoV-2 (COVID-19) struck. And as we all know, it lasted much longer than SARS-CoV. The funny thing is, SARS-CoV is actually deadlier than SARS-CoV-2, but SARS-CoV-2 spreads faster and farther, which is why it turned into a global pandemic and has killed so many more people (approximately 6.9 million at the time of this writing) than SARS-CoV. I talk more about what makes SARS-CoV-2 so contagious in the section "Understanding Why COVID-19 Is So Contagious," later in this chapter.

Transmitting and spotting SARS

SARS-CoV and SARS-CoV-2 are both airborne, which means you can catch it or spread it through coughing or sneezing, or coming into contact with infected saliva droplets. It also can live on surfaces, meaning if you touch a surface that someone who has SARS sneezed or coughed on, you can potentially pick those germs up on your hands. If you then touch your mouth, eyes, or nose without washing your hands, the virus can enter your system. (Flip to Chapter 5 if you want to read more on how people transmit COVID-19.)

If you get SARS, the first symptoms you notice are fever, headache, and body aches, which are pretty common among colds. You may think that these cold-like symptoms mean you have the common cold at first — but if you get sicker and the illness progresses to your respiratory system, you begin to recognize that you could have SARS. If you do have SARS-CoV or SARS-CoV-2, you might also have other symptoms. Table 2-1 shows a comparison of symptoms between colds and both SARS viruses.

REMEMBER

You can be asymptomatic and still have SARS-CoV or SARS-CoV-2.

TABLE 2-1 **Symptoms of Colds and SARS Viruses**

Symptoms	Common Cold	SARS CoV	SARS CoV-2 (COVID-19)
Body aches	✓	✓	✓
Fever		✓	✓
Headaches	✓	✓	✓
Diarrhea		✓	✓
Dry cough		✓	✓
Shortness of breath		✓	✓
Pneumonia		✓	✓
Loss of taste and/or smell			✓
Fatigue			✓
Runny nose	✓	✓	✓
Sore throat	✓	✓	✓
General malaise	✓	✓	✓

Distinguishing SARS-CoV and SARS-CoV-2

In addition to varying symptoms (which I talk about in the preceding section), you can find other differences between SARS–CoV and SARS–CoV–2. These include

>> **Incubation period:** For SARS-CoV, incubation takes 2 to 7 days, but SARS-CoV-2 can incubate from 1 to 14 days.

>> **Viral loads:** Although we don't know for sure yet, scientists believe that patients' upper respiratory tracts have greater amounts of the SARS-CoV-2 virus (know as *viral load*) than patients who have SARS-CoV. Although doctors are still researching the impacts of viral loads, they believe that the higher the viral load you have, the sicker you get, and the more likely you are to transmit the virus to others.

However, if you have SARS, you're much more likely to have symptoms soon after infection, which is why that original outbreak in 2003 was much easier to contain than COVID-19. During the SARS epidemic, symptomatic people isolated right away, serving to end the outbreak. If you become infected with COVID-19, you can have the virus for several days before symptoms occur. So during the early days of that epidemic in 2019, many COVID-positive, asymptomatic people didn't isolate, which is one of the biggest reasons why COVID-19 grew into the worldwide pandemic that it did.

Meeting MERS

Middle East Respiratory Syndrome (MERS) — just like SARS (see the section "Sizing up SARS," earlier in this chapter) — is both the virus and the illness. The distinction between terms is that MERS is the illness, and if you want to talk about the actual virus, it's MERS-CoV (Middle East Respiratory Syndrome Coronavirus).

MERS-CoV originated in Saudi Arabia in 2012. People typically contract the virus from dromedary camels, which explains why it's generally confined to that region of the world.

MERS has symptoms similar to SARS (fever, cough, shortness of breath, diarrhea, and pneumonia), but if you don't live in or haven't been to the Middle East lately, you probably can rule out MERS if you find yourself showing those symptoms.

Common cold variants

Within the coronavirus family are milder viruses that we've lived with for a very long time, such as 229E, NL63, OC43, and HKU1. They're often the cause of common cold symptoms, such as

>> Runny nose

>> Fever

>> Cough

>> Headache

>> Sore throat

>> General *malaise* (discomfort)

You can typically ride out or treat the symptoms easily by taking over-the-counter medications, hydrating yourself, and resting. Even if the illness progresses to bronchitis or pneumonia, you still can usually recover pretty well after you receive the proper treatment.

TIP

If you don't get better after a few days of experiencing cold symptoms — or certainly if you experience chills or body aches, or get worse in other ways — COVID-19 is a possibility. Test for the COVID-19 virus, either at home or with a medical professional. If you need more info on testing, flip to Chapter 7.

Meeting the COVID-19 Variants

COVID-19 is a determined enemy. No matter what the medical community comes up with to treat and prevent it, this virus finds a way forward. Viruses naturally evolve and mutate in order to overcome the obstacles placed in their way (such as natural antibodies and vaccines), and COVID-19 is no different.

What virus variants do

Virus mutations initially occur randomly, but the ones that help the virus to evade our immune responses also enable the resulting strains of the virus to multiply better and thrive. Every time SARS-CoV-2 mutates in a way that enhances its survival, the virus creates a *variant* — a slightly new strain or version of itself. The World Health Organization (WHO) monitors and identifies new variants. When a new variant emerges, the WHO names it by using the Greek alphabet, and researchers in the health community study these new variants in hopes of discovering how to treat and vaccinate against them.

Since the pandemic began in 2020, the COVID-19 virus has experienced multiple variants, which all behave differently. I don't list all of them in detail here because the difference between some variants is marginal. Besides, by the time this book goes to print, people will probably have at least one more variant to face. So for now, the following section looks at the two most common variants.

The most well-known variants: Delta and Omicron

Delta and Omicron are probably the most well-known COVID-19 variants to date:

>> **Delta:** This variant surfaced in 2020 and seemed even more infectious than previous variants. From Delta, the medical community discovered that humanity needs to employ multiple methods of prevention that reduce the spread of the virus — such as vaccines, social distancing, ventilation, masks, isolation of people with the disease, and quarantine of those who are exposed.

At the time of writing, the general population isn't in the midst of Delta infections anymore, but even if you're vaccinated, wearing a mask and keeping your distance whenever you feel a bit under the weather (or you're around someone else who does) help everyone stay safe.

>> **Omicron:** Omicron came around in November 2021. It was more contagious than the variants before it and gave rise to the most transmissible strains seen yet. Scientists theorize that it's so transmissible because most of Omicron's mutations live on the spike proteins, and those mutations are twice as infectious as the original spike proteins (see the section "Examining coronavirus structure" earlier in this chapter). The Omicron variants also result in a less severe disease than those that preceded them. Omicron is an example of a virus that has evolved into a form that's more contagious, but it doesn't often kill the host.

Mutating to a contagious, less deadly form is the best way for a virus to survive. The original Omicron strain is now gone, but its variants continue to impact us. Currently, your best weapon against the Omicron variant is receiving the bivalent booster shots (find out more about vaccines and boosters in Chapter 6).

Understanding Why COVID-19 Is So Contagious

Although COVID-19 continues to evolve through variants (flip back to "Meeting the COVID-19 Variants," earlier in this chapter, for more on variants), its impact seems to be weakening. People aren't getting as sick as they were in the beginning of the pandemic. Symptoms are milder and more treatable. This shift to milder symptoms is thanks — in large part — to vaccines (see the section "Surveying the Science of Vaccines," later in this chapter.)

But COVID-19 is still a real concern, so don't get complacent. Other factors keep the illness alive and moving through the population.

Less effective antibodies

White blood cells produce antibodies that fight off illnesses. Antibodies are attuned to specific viruses or bacteria, meaning COVID-19 antibodies can fight off only the COVID-19 virus. They can't fight off, say, an influenza virus (which causes the flu). And here's the added rub: Many antibodies aren't only virus-specific, but also variant-specific. As a result, the antibodies that protected you against the first COVID variant may not protect you as well against other variants.

Although having antibodies against a different strain of the same virus may not prevent you from getting that virus or transmitting it to others, those antibodies can protect you from severe illness because they can still slow down the ability of the virus to reproduce. This means fewer viruses will be present, making the disease less severe.

The variants are nature's way of keeping the virus alive. Each variant is slightly different in order to help the virus beat the antibodies that you develop after actually getting COVID or receiving the vaccine. And so, people are still getting COVID-19 now, even though several years have elapsed since the beginning of the pandemic. When Omicron hit, researchers found that our antibodies were only partially effective to fight it off, which is why it was such a fast-and-furious spreader at first.

WHY DON'T SOME PEOPLE GET COVID?

Despite the fact that the Omicron variant is so contagious, many of us know of someone who has never gotten COVID-19. Although we don't know the reason for sure, it may be because these people don't have the structure in their respiratory tract to which the virus attaches.

Spreading silently

One of the main reasons COVID-19 spreads like wildfire is that an infected person becomes contagious days before showing symptoms. And because you spread the virus through actions such as regular coughing and sneezing (if you want to read more on how you transmit COVID-19, flip to Chapter 5), you can be out and about on the town one day, feeling fine without a care in the world — but you're spreading COVID-19 to everyone around you, unbeknownst to you.

By the time you realize that you actually feel sick, it's too late — you've already had many interactions with other people while you were contagious. You've already spread the virus, and it's well on its way to affecting everyone you came in contact with yesterday, as well as those you're in contact with now.

Surveying the Science of Vaccines

In order to fight off *pathogens* (the scientific word for germs that cause disease), your immune system creates antibodies. Your immune system also has white blood cells that can attack invaders. Your body naturally overcomes a cold, flu, or other sickness by using these antibodies and white blood cells. And if those defenses aren't enough, your immune system also has memory white blood cells, which remember a previous infection (such as chickenpox) and get called into action if such an invader tries to attack you again.

But sometimes, your body just can't create the right type of or enough antibodies to fight off an illness because your immune system has never seen that pathogen before. In this case, you can benefit from taking a vaccine that can help prevent infection in the first place.

Knowing how vaccines work

Scientists take small parts of infectious organisms — a piece of the pathogen — and combine them with a carrier fluid to make up a vaccine that doctors can then inject into your body. Scientists can take these parts from real but modified viruses or bacteria or from a lab-manufactured version of the germ. Vaccines can also be made from live pathogens which have been modified so that they cannot cause disease.

What's key about vaccines is that they contain a form of the virus that doesn't cause disease but still prompts your body to generate an immune response. After you receive the vaccine injection, your body responds to the infection, figures out how to fight it off, and creates a blueprint so that it can remember how to fight if that same pathogen shows up again.

REMEMBER

Technically, the viruses aren't alive because they cannot reproduce without a host.

Needing one or more vaccine injections

With some vaccines, it's one-and-done, such as the chicken pox injection (although a vaccine for that didn't exist when I was growing up). Some vaccines (such as for the flu) are given annually — so you go every year and get a vaccine that's been slightly adjusted to deal with that particular year's strain. Some vaccines have multiple doses, so you need several shots weeks or months apart.

For the vaccines that are one-and-done, the related virus doesn't change much, so your immunity induced by a vaccine or natural infection remains effective. The protection that you receive from the vaccines for these little-changing germs is lifelong, and you don't have to get repeated vaccines. For diseases such as influenza and COVID-19, the virus changes, so the immunity induced by previous strains (either from natural infection or vaccination) doesn't completely protect you against being infected by new strains. So for changeable pathogens, scientists have to develop new vaccines that contain the new strains, and you need to receive these new vaccinations to retain immunity.

No vaccines of any kind can give you COVID-19 or any infection. Because your body can sometimes take a few weeks to create its battle blueprint, you can potentially contract the virus before you're fully protected, therefore getting sick. But that's a matter of terrible coincidental timing and isn't the vaccine's fault.

Varieties of COVID-19 vaccines

No matter whether you get one or multiple doses, all vaccines give your body a memory to draw from when it comes time to do battle against the illness. The FDA has approved for use in the United States three kinds of vaccines for COVID-19: mRNA, protein sub-unit, and viral vector.

mRNA

Messenger ribonucleic acid (mRNA) is a molecule that tells your body to make proteins, and mRNA vaccines contain mRNA that's made in a lab. After the vaccine enters your body, your muscle cells create the spike protein that replicates the mRNA from the vaccine. Then, the body breaks down the mRNA immediately after it is used to make protein. The mRNA from the vaccine never enters your cells' nuclei, where your DNA is, nor otherwise remains intact in your system. In the meantime, your body realizes the spike protein is an intruder and mounts an attack.

Scientists develop mRNA vaccines to protect against not only COVID-19, but also the flu, Zika virus, and rabies. These vaccines may even be used in some cancer treatments. Currently, the available mRNA vaccines for COVID-19 are made by Pfizer-BioNTech, and Moderna. In the future, companies may produce mRNA vaccines that protect against many pathogens at the same time, thus reducing the number of shots that children need to receive for preventative care. Many traditional vaccines — such as MMR — protect against more than one disease (in this case, measles, mumps, and rubella). The mRNA vaccine technology may enable scientists to combine protection against many more diseases into one vaccine.

Protein subunit

Protein subunit vaccines contain only certain pieces of the spike protein, which trigger your body to create antibodies and white blood cells. Currently, Novavax makes a protein subunit COVID-19 vaccination. It's a little tricky to understand the difference between this and mRNA, but basically, the protein subunit vaccine contains a protein from the virus itself, which is different from the spike protein protrusions from the virus body.

Viral vector

Viral vector vaccines use a virus that's not pathogenic to deliver deoxyribonucleic acid (DNA). DNA is in all of your cells and carries the genetic information, which leads to the production of the proteins that your body uses for development and basic functioning. Your cells use this DNA to make mRNA, which is then used to make proteins. The vaccine only includes DNA which produces the specific mRNA, which then builds out the spike protein. That spike protein, in turn, causes an immune response to SARS CoV-2.

IN THIS CHAPTER

» **Beginning in Wuhan, China**

» **Lagging behind in preventive measures**

» **Seeing COVID-19 spread around the world**

» **Responding as a global community**

» **Managing information and the new normal**

Chapter **3**

Examining the 2019 Global Pandemic

The COVID-19 pandemic was one of the most influential global events of modern times. It changed the flow of life (as we know it) — in some ways, permanently — and raised our awareness of the potential for untimely death around the world. It changed how governments administer and manage public health. It changed how individuals take care of themselves and each other. It even changed how business and enterprise (and the employees within those organizations) operate. Although the World Health Organization (WHO) declared the initial pandemic over on May 5, 2023, COVID-19's impact remains wide-reaching and affects nearly every corner of the globe.

In this chapter, I give you an overview of the history of one of the most significant global health crises in recent history. I take you from the first inklings of trouble — in Wuhan, China in late 2019 — and lead you through the fierce global spread throughout 2020 and 2021.

Looking at Where It Began: Wuhan, China

Although evidence (from research such as "Dating first cases of COVID-19," by David L. Roberts and others, published by plos. org on June 24, 2021: https://doi.org/10.1371/journal. ppat.1009620) points to cases of a mysterious illness starting as early as October or November of 2019, the first real cluster of cases presented itself in December of 2019. At that time, a group of patients in Wuhan, China experienced symptoms such as shortness of breath and fever. The symptoms were similar to those of pneumonia, but the patients didn't improve with standard treatments.

While the disease spread rapidly within Wuhan and other parts of China, the Chinese Center for Disease Control and Prevention (China CDC) started investigating the virus in-depth. Also, the World Health Organization (WHO) became involved and determined that the virus was a coronavirus, and likely a new strain of Severe Acute Respiratory Syndrome (SARS; see Chapter 2), which caused an outbreak of serious illness in China from 2002 to 2004.

Marketplace, lab, or somewhere else

The WHO investigation found that most of the original patients in Wuhan in 2019 had been in direct or indirect contact with the Huanan Seafood Wholesale Market. This discovery narrowed in on the market as *ground zero* (the starting point or base) for the virus. WHO officials and other agencies needed to investigate further, but while cases began to grow, authorities in Wuhan closed the market and refused to share information about the market or grant investigative access to virtually all people. This stonewalling made it difficult — if not impossible — for the world to gather much-needed data about the virus and understand as much as possible, as quickly as possible.

After the first reports of the live animal market hit the media, scientists theorized that animals (specifically, horseshoe bats) in the market had a virus that they somehow transmitted to humans (a phenomenon called *zoonotic spillover*). But scientists had difficulty proving the theory because Wuhan authorities had already removed all animals from the market, cleaned it, and closed it. These actions made it impossible for scientists to find test specimens or to gather data.

In the Huanan Seafood Wholesale Market, many different living species of animals existed closely together with humans for extended periods of time. This kind of environment provides the perfect place for a zoonotic virus to spill over. Placing a live animal market in the middle of a large population center, rather than in a remote area, further increases the chance for such a virus to develop. To find out more about how and why zoonotic viruses transmit to humans, flip to Chapter 2.

Without confirmation that the first humans contracted the SAR-CoV-2 virus (which causes COVID-19) while in the market, the public and medical communities around the world began to develop other theories. For example, some sources said that the virus was accidentally released from the nearby Wuhan Institute of Virology, or that the U.S. or China deliberately released the virus as a bioweapon. Another theory claimed that China knew the outbreak was happening much earlier than it publicly admitted.

Studies that suggest the marketplace as the source

Major studies from July 2022 strongly suggest that the source of the COVID-19 virus was indeed the Huanan Seafood Wholesale Market, and not the result of release or leakage from a lab. These studies include:

>> **A failed-attempts study:** This study, led by Jonathan Pekar, a Ph.D. candidate in biomedical informatics at the University of California San Diego, which was published in the journal *Science* (Vol 377, Issue 6609), explains that viruses often make multiple failed attempts before they succeed in jumping to humans. In this case, initial reports of illnesses suggest that two early lineages of COVID-19 were probably transmitted from animals to humans in November through December 2019.

>> **Genetic analysis and geolocation studies:** Two other studies — authored by Michael Worobey, an evolutionary biologist at the University of Arizona, and others — were also published in the journal *Science* (Vol 377, Issue 6609). These studies show how the Huanan market was almost certainly the epicenter of the outbreak, based on geolocations and genetic analysis of the virus.

Add these findings to the multiple known cases of a virus transmitting the other way — from humans to animals, in the instance of influenza or measles, for example — and a zoonotic spillover became the most plausible theory.

Support for non-marketplace origins

Not all authorities agree that zoonotic spillover is the most likely explanation. As recently as February 2023, the U.S. Department of Energy's intelligence agency said (with *low confidence*, which means it's possible, but not probable) that it believed the virus originated from a lab leak. Some key points in the lab leak theory include

>> The China National Accreditation Service for Conformity Assessment (CNAS) certified Wuhan Institute of Virology (WIV) as the first lab in China to handle the most dangerous pathogens in the world, and scientists at WIV conducted the first research on coronaviruses found in bats.

>> Three lab workers from WIV reportedly sought medical treatment in November 2019, according to a U.S. intelligence report that the *Wall Street Journal* gained access to.

>> Chinese doctor Li Wenliang tried to warn the medical community about a possible outbreak in December 2019 after he'd seen seven patients for SARS-CoV-2. To silence him, his hospital censured him and the Chinese government made him sign a document stating he lied and spread false information. He died of COVID-19 in February 2020.

The lack of information from the early days of the COVID-19 virus pandemic made it next to impossible to ever know its true source. Even today, we still struggle to understand its origin — but most scientists and other experts agree that the likeliest explanation has the virus jumping from animals to humans in the marketplace.

Delays in Recognition and Response

While the cases of COVID-19 in China grew, the rest of the world watched but didn't understand the severity of the outbreak for a couple of reasons:

>> **Lack of information:** Because China remained intentionally obtuse with their information and reporting, its own citizens — and even the governments of other countries — had difficulty ascertaining how serious and wide-reaching this outbreak was and would become.

>> **Lack of response:** Also, the WHO didn't activate quickly enough to declare COVID-19 a pandemic and advise governments to shut down their industries. This too-little-too-late approach was another major contributing factor that caused a delayed and inadequate response to the pandemic.

These factors allowed COVID-19 to spread far and fast before the global population truly understood that COVID-19 was a major health threat around the world (find more about the threat and response in the section "Watching the Virus Spread Globally," later in this chapter).

In the earliest weeks and months of the pandemic, constantly changing information from news and medical-community sources and confusion on the part of government officials ruled the day. The rest of the world watched in disbelief. The horrendous initial response to recommendations that people take preventative measures seriously, especially in the U.S., frankly didn't get much better for some time. Even after the WHO and the CDC formed local and global messages (that COVID-19 cases were spreading beyond China and that SARS-CoV-2 is a highly contagious and potentially deadly virus), many people remained uncertain. For example, some people

>> **Didn't believe COVID-19 was a real threat:** They believed it was nothing more than a common flu or cold, and that either the number of deadly cases was exaggerated, people with COVID-19 were dying of something else, or only people with other serious illnesses were getting very sick from COVID-19.

>> **Believed that the entire concept of a pandemic was made up and that the virus didn't exist.** We in the medical community encountered people dying of COVID-19 who still insisted that they didn't have it and that the pandemic was a hoax.

Because COVID-19 was novel to the medical community, spokes-people, governments, and health agencies had to figure out what was going on while the outbreak unfolded. This situation led to rapidly-changing insights and reports that often gave conflict-ing information about prevention, transmission, hot spots, and the capacity of various countries' healthcare infrastructure. Con-flicting viewpoints led the people who doubted whether COVID-19 was real to further disbelieve what they heard from authorities.

Watching the Virus Spread Globally

By January 2020, COVID-19 spread beyond Wuhan because infected individuals traveled, unknowingly carrying the virus with them, and leading to localized outbreaks in other cities and countries.

Identifying cases outside of China

Outside of Wuhan, COVID-19 first spread to countries that had close ties to China — such as the Republic of Korea, Japan, and Thailand — in January 2020. Shortly after reports of this spread occurred, the U.S. CDC started screening travelers on flights to and from selected high-risk hubs.

Confirming how COVID-19 was spreading

While more cases emerged that didn't tie directly to the seafood market — and even showed up in other countries altogether — it became more and more apparent that COVID-19 was spread-ing from human to human. Scientists, doctors, and independent research groups worked together worldwide and shared their findings to understand how COVID-19 was moving.

The WHO also convened a global study on the origin of the virus that included scientists from various countries, as well as WHO's own health emergencies personnel. Together, these experts stud-ied the virus's epidemiology, genetic sequences, and the human-animal interface component to confirm that human-to-human transmission was occurring and better understand the virus's origins.

By January 2020, the WHO confirmed that humans can transmit COVID-19, and Dr. Zhong Nanshan, a prominent scientist in China, was one of the first to confirm this in a state television interview on January 20, 2020. This discovery was a critical moment and, after this confirmation, Wuhan locked down on January 23, 2020. But cases outside of Wuhan already existed, and the virus spread rapidly.

COVID infections and deaths sweep the globe

Because international and domestic travelling remained mostly intact (except for a few high-risk hubs), transmissions around the world increased rapidly and resulted in severe disease cases and fatalities. The first COVID-19 death in Wuhan was on January 11, 2020, and by February 10, 2020, over 1,000 were dead worldwide from COVID-19.

People who had pre-existing health conditions (including the elderly) were hit extra hard. Thousands developed severe symptoms — most notably, acute respiratory distress. Hospitals around the world maxed out with COVID-19 patients (many of whom required intensive care).

REMEMBER

The World Health Organization (WHO) declared COVID-19 a global pandemic on March 11, 2020. By then, the virus had infected more than 118,000 people and caused over 4,200 deaths worldwide.

Tracking the Response to the Pandemic

As soon as the WHO declared the global pandemic, nations and governments around the world fought to contain the spread of the virus and treat people soon after infection — before they got too severely ill (or died). The initial months of the pandemic filled people with uncertainty and fear. They perceived that the medical community still knew very little about COVID-19 and couldn't seem to stop it. The disease raged like wildfire around the world.

WHO: Taking charge around the world

The World Health Organization (WHO) played a key role in the global response to the COVID-19 pandemic from the disease's early stages, fulfilling its mission to direct and coordinate international health within the United Nations system. Overall, the public opinion about how the WHO handled COVID-19 is mixed, with some people believing that the organization did a great job (all things considered), and others believing that they should have done more to alleviate the pandemic.

REMEMBER

The WHO works primarily as an advisory body, providing guidelines, collecting data, and coordinating global efforts, but it doesn't have enforcement power. Enforcing guidelines and best practices to stop the spread of COVID-19 fell to governments.

Taking early actions

In the early days of the pandemic, WHO followed the actions outlined in Table 3-1 to investigate and devise a response to the influence of COVID-19.

TABLE 3-1 The WHO COVID-19 Response

Action	When	Result
Initial response	January 5, 2020	Notification to the world via the WHO disease outbreak news platform regarding cases of pneumonia of unknown cause in Wuhan, China on December 31, 2019
Wuhan field visit and investigation	January 20–21, 2020	Confirmation that COVID-19 is transmissible between humans
Public health emergency declaration	January 30, 2020	A Public Health Emergency of International Concern (PHEIC) alarm, the highest level WHO can use under international law to mobilize resources
Global pandemic declaration	March 11, 2020	Announcement at a news briefing that the COVID-19 outbreak was a pandemic

Continuing with pandemic guidance

After declaring COVID-19 a pandemic on March 11, 2020, the WHO took further action to guide the public through the pandemic, including

>> **Providing health and safety guidelines and recommendations** so that countries could control the spread of the

virus. Examples included social distancing, hand hygiene, masking, testing, treatment, and isolation of patients.

>> **Providing support, supplies, and training to countries,** especially those that had weaker health systems. This support included personal protective equipment (PPE) and diagnostic tests. The WHO also hosted virtual training for healthcare workers.

>> **Coordinating global efforts to develop testing and treatment,** including vaccines. The WHO's Solidarity Trial assessed the effectiveness of different drug treatments. And in partnership with the Global Alliance for Vaccines and Immunization (GAVI), and the Coalition for Epidemic Preparedness Innovations (CEPI), WHO established the *COVAX initiative*, which helped to accelerate development and production of COVID-19 tests, treatments, and vaccines. The initiative also helped to ensure that lower-GDP countries had access to vaccines when those vaccines became approved.

>> **Regularly collecting and sharing data about cases, symptoms, and deaths.** The WHO was at the forefront, providing real-time updates on all virus developments. They also hosted an online tool that tracked the global spread of the virus (which is still active as of the time of writing, but not updated as regularly).

Making some missteps

Although the essential actions outlined in Table 3-1 and the preceding section drove the response to the pandemic in the right direction, the WHO made several missteps that planted seeds of doubt and decreased the public's confidence in the WHO's guidance. For example

>> **Delaying their declarations:** Many members of the public, health officials, and members of the medical community think that the WHO was too slow in declaring COVID-19 first a PHEIC and then a pandemic, and if they had made those declarations earlier, far fewer people would have died.

>> **Sharing contradictory information on human-to-human transmission:** Based on the information it had at the time, the WHO initially stated on January 14, 2020, that there was "no clear evidence of human-to-human transmission," but on January 19, 2020, after they received additional information

from the Japanese Ministry of Health, Labour, and Welfare and the Pan American Health Organization, they had to correct themselves just five days later.

>> **Not restricting travel soon enough:** In February 2020, the WHO advised against travel restrictions to and from China, but many health officials believe this advice was a mistake because it allowed the unchecked spread of COVID-19 to continue around the world.

>> **Failing to independently verify data:** Government officials and members of the medical community also argue that the WHO relied too much on information provided by China in the early stages of the outbreak, leading to misinformation (or inadequate information) about the severity and transmission of the illness.

>> **Giving confusing masking guidance:** Early in the pandemic, the WHO advised against the general public wearing masks unless they were sick or caring for someone who was sick. And they didn't change their guidance to suggest that everyone wear masks until June 2020. Failing to guide the public to mask earlier perpetuated the spread.

REMEMBER

Hindsight is 20/20. Despite their mistakes, the WHO had to act within constantly changing and evolving circumstances. They often had access to limited data and had to decide what to share and when to share it, balancing the importance of informing the public with not panicking them.

CDC: Directing the U.S.'s response

The U.S. Centers for Disease Control and Prevention (CDC), the national public health agency of the United States, played a significant role in managing and responding to the COVID-19 pandemic. Much like the WHO (see the section "WHO: Taking charge around the world," earlier in this chapter), they collected and disseminated data, developed and implemented guidelines for public health and safety, and facilitated testing and vaccine distribution.

Public opinion of the CDC's handling of the pandemic varied widely. On the one hand, their guidance became the cornerstone of the medical community's virus management strategies and public health practices. On the other hand, they — like the WHO — often didn't act quickly enough to stop the pandemic before it started, gave out conflicting information, or didn't execute initiatives effectively (for example, when CDC leadership rejected offers from their lab technicians to work extra hours to help in the early days of the pandemic).

During the pandemic, the CDC

>> **Created and maintained updated COVID-19 data online,** including case numbers, hospitalizations, and deaths on a national and state level.

>> **Conducted research,** such as studying where and how the virus originated, how the virus is spread, the effectiveness of masking, and of treatments and vaccines when they became available.

>> **Developed and updated public health and safety guidelines** for businesses, schools, healthcare facilities, and the general public. Unfortunately, at times, the CDC gave inconsistent messaging, especially about masking and transmission.

>> **Developed and distributed COVID-19 diagnostic tests;** however, the public criticized them for widespread delays, shortfall of supply, and less-than-impressive test accuracy when they first made the tests available to the public.

>> **Provided guidelines for vaccine distribution and administration,** prioritizing healthcare workers and the elderly.

>> **Maintained current updates about vaccination rates and efficacy,** which allowed governments and health agencies around the world to know how well the vaccines and treatments were working, as well as when to lift travel and isolation mandates, for example.

REMEMBER

To be fair, the CDC had to study and respond to a new virus in real-time. But because the general public doesn't have much experience with how rapidly information about viruses can change, resulting in frequent changes in recommendations, the public often felt confused, frustrated, distrustful, and exhausted. These feelings left significant portions of the public reluctant to follow the most current guidelines, or they decided to give up following any guidelines at all.

Because the pandemic was such constant and far-reaching news, some U.S. media outlets and politicians took the opportunity to politicize the CDC's (and the WHO's) guidance, leading to further divisions in public opinion.

DR FAUCI: THE FACE OF THE U.S. RESPONSE

During the COVID-19 response, Dr. Anthony Fauci was the Director of the National Institute of Allergy and Infectious Diseases (NIAID), and he became the face of the U.S. response to the COVID-19 pandemic in many ways. Much of the public immediately appreciated his calm demeanor and trusted his experience.

He brought years of expertise to the table, could communicate complicated and frightening concepts in easy-to-understand ways, and was unrelenting in his availability. Dr Fauci regularly appeared in press conferences, interviews, talk shows, and more, always providing updates and sharing his expertise on the evolving situation. He was honest and transparent, not afraid to tell the public that he didn't know something, and willing to stand firm when he knew without a doubt what the right practice was. The way he addressed the public didn't seem like a marketer or spin doctor; to most people, he felt like their friendly primary care physician who truly invested himself in the best outcome.

Additionally, throughout the pandemic, Dr. Fauci consistently advocated for science. He always brought his answers to any questions or concerns back to the evidence he had at the time. He carefully considered what researchers knew to be true when directing public policy.

However, not everyone liked him. For example, Dr. Fauci faced plenty of critics and backlash during the pandemic on what some thought was flip-flopping. For example, he (along with the CDC and WHO, to be fair) initially advised against the public masking because he wanted to prevent shortages for healthcare workers. When the evidence started showing how effectively masking could prevent the spread of COVID-19, Dr. Fauci changed his guidance, making many members of the public distrustful. The same thing happened when Dr. Fauci changed his guidelines around reopening after federal, state, and local governments shut down all non-essential businesses. By then, large portions of the population had politicized him because he often publicly contradicted messaging from government officials who (knowingly or unknowingly) spread misinformation.

Overall, Dr. Fauci served the pandemic well, but he wasn't without mistakes or controversy. Despite efforts by some members of the public to politicize those few mistakes amongst his many episodes of speaking truth to power, the great majority of experts in infectious diseases (including me) regard Dr. Anthony Fauci as a hero.

State and local government shutdowns

While COVID-19 cases continued to rise in the United States in the early months of 2020, the U.S. government's Coronavirus Task Force gave general suggestions for shutdown and other public mandates, but did not enforce them, leaving that task to the state governments instead. For example, states decided how to handle

>> **Shutdowns:** Each state developed and enforced their own shutdown mandates, with many shutting down schools, restaurants, bars, gyms, and entertainment venues first, while limiting the size of group gatherings elsewhere. The shutdowns then spilled over to all non-essential businesses.

>> **Orders to stay home:** Most states issued stay-at-home or shelter-in-place orders, which meant all citizens had to stay home, unless they were essential workers, such as health-care providers, law enforcement, utilities workers, and employees of food stores, pharmacies, and liquor stores.

>> **Social distancing:** When people had to leave their homes, state governments often mandated that they keep a minimum of 6 feet of social distance between themselves and others — and wear a mask.

Differing state and national responses

Although some states had very strong and long shutdowns, others had shorter or less strict mandates, depending on

>> The severity of the outbreak in different areas

>> Varying interpretations of the guidance coming from the CDC, the WHO, and government officials

>> The need for economic stability

>> Political affiliations

Table 3-2 offers a look back at how the shutdowns and stay-at-home orders rolled out across the U.S. in 2020.

TABLE 3-2 COVID-19 Recommendations in 2020

When	By Whom	What
March 15	CDC	Recommends cancelling all in-person events that consist of 50 or more people for eight weeks
March 16	White House Coronavirus Task Force	Recommends avoiding social gatherings of more than 10 people, or eating or drinking at bars, restaurants, and food courts, for two weeks to *flatten the curve* (reduce the rate of increase in COVID cases)
March 19	California	Implements a statewide stay-at-home order
March 21	New York, Illinois, and Connecticut	Implement statewide stay-at-home orders
April 1	Florida and Texas	Implement stay-at-home orders
April 2	At least 38 states, the District of Columbia, and Puerto Rico	Implement some form of stay-at-home order
April 16	White House Coronavirus Task Force	Releases guidelines to help state and local officials reopen
May	All states	Lift stay-at-home orders and gradually reopen businesses and public spaces (specific protocols and timelines vary widely between states)
Fall and winter	Some states	Reactivate selected restrictions when cases spike again

Less-than-collaborative responses to pandemic restrictions

Because emotions were so high during the pandemic to begin with, the different policies from state to state (and even city to city) often created tension and controversy among the public — and even officials — who tried to balance public health with economic needs. For example

>> **Public officials refused to implement guidelines.** The governors of Florida and South Dakota refused to implement statewide masking and other mandates, even as the number of COVID-19 cases in their states increased.

>> **People protested in the streets.** Michigan residents protested the governor's stay-at-home orders at the state capitol, saying the mandates were infringing on their freedom. Similar protests occurred in Wisconsin, Ohio, and North Carolina.

>> **Masking policies became a particularly heated issue**, with different states, cities, and businesses handling masking in their own ways. Some individuals and businesses also openly defied shutdown orders or mask mandates, resulting in legal battles and heightened tension within communities.

Not only did inconsistent policies confuse and frustrate the public, but those inconsistencies also highly politicized masking, with people choosing to patronize businesses based on their masking policies. In some cases, confrontations over mask requirements even turned violent.

REMEMBER

Although violence is never the answer to problems, the driving force behind this violence was usually fear of losing income and financial stability. Small businesses got hit especially hard, with state governments telling mom-and-pop shops that they had to close, while allowing big box stores to remain open. For many people, the inconsistent shutdowns seemed unfair and totally fatal to their financial well-being. Many businesses never recovered.

Public information and education campaigns

During the COVID-19 pandemic, many people constantly looked to TV news, radio shows, sources of information on the Internet, newspapers, and even friends and family, because they wanted to get the latest pandemic updates. Because the shutdowns meant that most people couldn't go out, and they wanted the latest updates on constantly-changing information, international and domestic public education campaigns from different agencies and officials became an integral part of most people's daily lives.

The CDC led many of these campaigns at the federal level, providing

>> Current, scientifically sourced information about symptoms, testing, and prevention

>> Reports about case and death numbers

>> Educational and news resources in many languages for different audiences, including the general public, healthcare professionals, schools, businesses, and community organizations

States and cities also launched their own campaigns to report on local cases and mandates, mirroring the federal effort by disseminating information through websites, social media, television, and radio, and even by text message. Yet, at times, the information from different levels of government officials and agencies contradicted each other, again frustrating the public and fostering distrust and skepticism.

Still, some campaigns successfully communicated simple and consistent messaging that helped people stay informed and healthy, such as

>> **#StayHome:** Many organizations and celebrities endorsed this social media campaign that encouraged people to stay home and practice social distancing in order to slow the spread of the virus.

>> **#Masks4All:** This social media campaign encouraged people to use cloth masks in public and gave resources for crafting homemade masks, highlighting how research by the U.S. CDC had shown masks could help stop COVID-19 from spreading.

>> **Science in 5:** The WHO launched a series of videos and articles that explained the science behind COVID-19 in an easy-to-understand manner.

>> **How to Protect Yourself and Others:** This online resource from the CDC provided clear, concise guidelines about hand hygiene, social distancing, mask wearing, and what to do if you become ill.

These and other campaigns raised awareness about COVID-19 and helped keep the public as safe as possible — in addition to ending the pandemic as soon as possible.

Walking the Too-Much-Information Line

While the COVID-19 pandemic took hold and the public stayed glued to devices to avoid missing a minute of the 24-hour news cycle, people found it more and more difficult to stay informed without succumbing to unfounded panic or fear.

The constant flow of conflicting or alarming updates challenged many people's ability to manage their anxiety and stay rational. With reports of terrible sickness and death all around, so many people felt desperate to stay safe (and keep friends and families safe).

Controlling information intake

In a time when so much felt out of a single person's control, knowledge was one thing everyone could have power over — you could consume as much news as possible. And for many, information was the best and only weapon against the pandemic.

But you (and everyone else) had to walk a delicate line between remaining knowledgeable about the evolving situation and spiraling into an abyss of information overload that could lead to distress and hysteria.

In order to stay sane, some people had to create boundaries for themselves, such as turning off the TV or avoiding the Internet for a certain amount of time each day. As a healthcare worker myself, I had to make sure I had the most current information, but I also needed to remain steady and calm so that I could do my best work and help as much as possible. In fact, I spent time listening to sports radio to lessen the COVID-19 information overload.

The pandemic's 24-hour news cycle shifted the public's news consumption habits significantly. People tuned in multiple times a day to get the latest updates on the virus's spread, the discoveries about it, government mandates and assistance programs, and more. This urgent (and borderline obsessive) level of engagement with news — which people all around the world felt — was unprecedented for a situation unprecedented in most people's memory.

The media consumption balance

Trying to keep the public informed but not incite massive panic challenged media outlets at all levels. On one hand, public health authorities and government officials had to communicate the seriousness of the pandemic and the importance of complying with safety measures. On the other hand, they didn't want to cause panic responses among the public, such as hoarding supplies or rebelling against the guidance offered.

During this time, mental health professionals encouraged people to try their best to balance their one-way media consumption with activities that kept them grounded as human beings. Many people found following this advice challenging during isolation, quarantines, and lockdowns — but people who maintained routines, connected with loved ones, and took breaks from the news typically stayed healthier and happier than those who didn't.

Deciphering travel limitations

People had trouble keeping up with the constant stream of updates on travel advisories, border closures, flight cancellations, and quarantine regulations. Even though the WHO, the CDC, and various governments shut down non-essential travel at various times and to varying degrees, people still needed to travel during the pandemic for essential reasons, such as deaths in the family or other emergencies. Those who traveled during this time faced a lot of stress for two distinct reasons:

>> People risked transmitting or contracting COVID-19 while traveling.

>> Guidelines changed very quickly and varied among potential destinations.

At the beginning of the pandemic, many people found themselves stranded outside of their home countries when airlines grounded their flights. Hundreds — if not thousands — faced this situation and had to figure out how to stay in non-native countries for months, unplanned. Some countries' embassies helped facilitate citizens getting back to their home countries, but others simply couldn't help because of inadequate resources and infrastructure.

Vying for customer service

Airlines and travel agencies were swamped with customers who needed service. The sheer volume of people needing assistance put tremendous pressure on these companies, leading to frustration and confusion for many customers. Travelers had to deal with unprecedented problems when trying to change or cancel travel plans, including incredibly long wait times to speak with customer services representatives across most, if not all, travel-based companies to get help with

- **Canceling or rebooking a trip:** With the sudden wave of cancellations and changes and limited numbers of available seats, customers had few options for changing their trips — and many couldn't even reach a live agent at all.

- **Vying for refunds and updated information:** Many people struggled to receive refunds for canceled trips, and they had to deal with often unclear or inconsistent information.

- **Winging it:** Travelers often had to book travel plans with partial information, just hoping the seat they booked existed, and that the flight (or train or bus trip) would actually depart.

Dealing with altered travel practices

At the same time, airlines and other travel companies needed to quickly implement new safety measures to protect the health of customers and employees, including deep cleaning, boarding- and deplaning-process changes, and new requirements for masks and other PPE.

Employees and passengers had to get used to the new policies (producing a negative COVID-19 test if flying into the US from an international location, for example) and practices (such as wearing masks), but after they did, it became second nature for most. And these changes improved other aspects of health and safety while traveling, for example by lowering the transmission of other communicable illnesses such as influenza.

REMEMBER

Even after the pandemic ended, many airlines still use some of the pandemic policies and procedures. For example, many airlines have kept their improved sanitation methods.

Tiptoeing into a New Normal

While the COVID-19 pandemic unfolded, people adopted new behaviors and habits. In 2018, most people didn't practice these habits regularly, but throughout 2020, people became experts at

- Social distancing
- Masking
- Frequent hand washing

>> Seeing (and using) hand sanitizer everywhere

>> Cleaning and disinfecting surfaces frequently

>> Being very aware of touching shared objects, surfaces, or our own faces

>> Using nods, waves, or elbow bumps by way of greeting, rather than handshakes

>> Attending virtual meetings and events

>> Conducting as many tasks as possible — for work, school, and shopping — virtually

>> Staying local and choosing outdoor locations for recreation

>> Quarantining after travel

At first, people treated most of these measures as temporary and tied directly to the pandemic. Because of all of the public campaigns and messaging, most people made these behaviors part of their daily routines. Although some of these practices (such as avoiding the gym) eventually ended when the pandemic ended, many of them (such as working remotely) are still part of the new normal.

Chapter **4**

Evaluating the Pandemic's Impact on Society

This world isn't the same as it was before the COVID-19 pandemic swept through. In many ways, the pandemic reshaped societal norms, economic structures, and international relations in ways that are likely permanent.

In addition to changes in personal hygiene and public health practices (see Chapter 3), people continue to feel the pandemic's effect on the economy and on business — particularly in sectors such as hospitality and travel, which don't have virtual equivalents. But some businesses thrived, if they could pivot to online models or other methods to meet changing needs and continue operation.

Although you can't easily predict any specific outcomes, you can clearly tell that the world after COVID-19 is (and will remain) different in many ways from the world that existed before the pandemic. This transformative moment offers both significant challenges and opportunities for change. In this chapter, you can find out details about the lasting effects of COVID-19 on not only health, but also lifestyle, business, work life, schooling, and nearly every aspect of our society.

Noting the Economic Fallout

The economic fallout of the pandemic, including high unemployment rates and economic recession, can shape economies and societies in the long term. The resulting changes can possibly lead to policy shifts and new approaches to social safety nets and economic stability. During the pandemic, the U.S. federal government, as well as state and local governments, enacted several measures to provide financial relief to people, including

>> **The Coronavirus Aid, Relief, and Economic Security (CARES) Act,** signed into law in March 2020. This bill included several key provisions, such as direct stimulus payments, expanded unemployment benefits, and eviction moratoriums.

>> **Financial aid packages** from many state and local governments. This unprecedented financial aid kept many individuals — who faced the hardship of lost jobs or reduced work hours — and their families afloat during the pandemic.

The reality of the devastating situation is that the economy has changed because of the pandemic, and many families have never truly recovered from the lost income and changed livelihoods.

Considering the Pandemic's Effects on Wellness

The pandemic's stay-at-home orders, gym closures, and general disruption of daily routines led people to significantly reduce their physical activity, becoming nearly sedentary in some cases. Many people spent long periods at home during lockdowns with not much to do.

In addition, the necessity for social distancing, quarantine, and isolation measures radically altered the dynamics of interpersonal interactions during the pandemic. These facts, along with the potential lasting health effects of having (and surviving) the COVID-19 virus, have left their mark on the general well-being of the world's population.

Loss of physical fitness

Because sports facilities, parks, and public rec areas — as well as gyms — all shut down, adults and children missed out on their regular sports activities, workouts, practices, and games. Simply staying active became more difficult, which was especially devastating to children (kids need to move!). Any parents of young children can attest to the cabin fever that seemed to set in almost immediately. (Am I right?) The parents had to get really creative with how they kept their kids moving, rather than sitting in front of the TV all day.

On top of not being able to get out and exercise as much, peoples' stress levels went up along with pandemic restrictions. And in some cases, dietary choices took an undesirable path while people sought out comfort or takeout foods. Because so many people were home all the time with nothing to do, many people chose to snack more, which — while delicious and comforting — came with weight gain and other drawbacks from processed foods (such as increased blood pressure, poor control of diabetes, and worsening of heart disease).

After the pandemic ended and everything fully opened again, many people returned to their old fitness routines and felt great, but others had (and have) to manage conditions such as diabetes, obesity, hypertension, or heart disease that came on (or got worse) during or after the pandemic.

Increased respiratory and cardiac events

One of COVID-19's major ongoing impacts is a significant increase in cardiac and respiratory events in people. In Chapter 9, I go into detail about these occurrences with my discussion of *Long COVID* (the condition where COVID-19 symptoms linger for weeks, months, or even years after recovering from the infection). Briefly, if you develop Long COVID or had a severe case of COVID-19, you may face the following health challenges:

» **Long-COVID:** The SARS-CoV-2 virus primarily affects the respiratory system, causing symptoms such as coughing, shortness of breath, and in severe cases, pneumonia. It can also cause permanent lung damage.

» **Severe COVID-19:** Some people who contracted a severe case of COVID-19 suffered from acute cardiac injury, which damages the heart muscle permanently and can lead to more serious complications, such as heart attacks, arrhythmias, and heart failure.

And as the paper "Perspective: cardiovascular disease and the Covid-19 pandemic" by Gori, Lelieveld, and Münzel (published in the April 10, 2020 issue of the journal *Basic Research in Cardiology*) indicates, hospitals have seen an increase in non-COVID-related cardiac events, possibly because some patients who had cardiac symptoms received delayed care, fearing that they would contract the virus by going to a medical facility. The long-term impact of these cardiac and respiratory events remains a major concern for post-COVID recovery.

A rise in social isolation and depression

During COVID-19 shutdowns and restrictions, many people were cut off from family, friends, and their wider social circles. Simultaneously, the abrupt end to attending school, the workplace, and social gatherings added to people feeling like they were absolutely marooned in their own homes.

During the height of the pandemic, very few people were on the streets — usually only essential workers or people making essential trips. When people had to go out, they made their excursions (to the drug store or supermarket, for example) quick and purposeful. Restrictions such as masking and social distancing didn't allow for lingering, so you couldn't ask those you encountered about how the kids are or what weekend plans they have.

Dealing with the lack of interaction

These quarantine and isolation conditions resulted in people becoming absolutely disconnected from each other, and many people were desperate for any type of human interaction. They resorted to phone calls, texts, and video conferencing for some type of interaction. *Zoom* (an online video-meeting tool) saw its usage increase exponentially when family and friend circles began to use it to host virtual gatherings.

Tools such as Zoom took the sting out of isolation, but seeing someone on a video call just still wasn't the same as being able to hug them. With no face-to-face interactions, on top of the constant cycle of distressing, confusing news and uncertainty, the world's collective stress and anxiety levels grew.

REMEMBER

Reports from the World Health Organization (WHO) demonstrate that more people became depressed during the pandemic. People who lived alone or in tense domestic environments, elderly individuals, and people who had pre-existing mental health conditions were particularly vulnerable to the onset or increase in poor mental health. Isolation and the loss of routine made so much of life feel hopeless and lonely for many people.

Gaining an awareness of mental health issues

The pandemic-related mental health crisis (touched on in the preceding section) does have a silver lining: Because so many people experienced mental health unwellness and crisis during the pandemic, more people now understand and respect the need for mental healthcare.

Companies have developed more app and web-based options for mental healthcare, and more people now access services such as teletherapy to get treated for their mental health conditions.

For children and adolescents, the pandemic presented unique restrictions and particularly challenging circumstances. According to WHO sources, many children

>> **Missed vital social development:** Especially if they were very young (under the age of 10), they now may feel disconnected from their peers, mentors, and even family members.

>> **Experienced (and are experiencing) heightened feelings of isolation, fear, and sadness:** These feelings result in depression and delayed development.

> » **Faced food insecurity, domestic violence, or parental unemployment conditions that they couldn't escape by going to school:** These situations have led to long-term physical and psychological effects (such as malnutrition, chronic illness, anxiety, aggression, and mental illness), the extent of which we don't yet fully know.

Increased substance abuse

During the pandemic, many people turned to substances (such as opioids like fentanyl and heroin, and stimulants like meth and cocaine) to help them deal with (or escape) stress, anxiety, and social isolation. And evidence of this turn to substances comes with the surge in alcohol sales, as reported by the NIH's National Institute on Alcohol Abuse and Alcoholism.

On top of that, people already dealing with substance abuse issues didn't have access to their regular support systems and recovery resources. Regular events, such as group therapy sessions and counseling, didn't happen because of social distancing and lockdowns. Many people in recovery relapsed in part because of the additional stress and lack of support. People could go days, weeks, even months without interacting in person, meaning someone could easily use or overuse a controlled or regulated substance, and no one knew to help.

THE IMPACT OF COVID-19 ON ASSISTED-LIVING COMMUNITIES

Assisted-living and retirement communities faced exceptionally difficult challenges during the pandemic. Because the population is so vulnerable to infection, in order to prevent outbreaks, staff had to enforce strict restrictions on visitation and group activities, often leading to prolonged isolation for their residents, which had devastating consequences, especially for patients with dementia and other cognitive decline.

In the early days of the pandemic, many facilities had inadequate personal protective equipment (PPE), testing, and infection control protocols. Staff implemented visitation policies to protect residents — but they often did so too late, after residents or employees already had COVID-19.

Many seniors were confined to their rooms alone without much, if any, interaction. Staff — who were prohibited in many cases from seeing patients face-to-face for fear of spreading COVID-19, plus extremely were overworked due to understaffing and illness in the ranks — brought them their meals individually. And if the residents had COVID-19, they were further isolated behind closed doors, not able to see other people at all. The impact of isolation on elderly patients, many of whom already had dementia, can't be overestimated. Without contact, many residents experienced profound loneliness and disconnection, which — in some cases — caused their decline and eventual death.

But the impossible-to-escape aspect of this isolation highlighted that many seniors are acutely aware of their vulnerability to sickness, and many residents in assisted living became truly afraid of catching COVID-19, especially if any of their neighbors became sick or died from the virus.

While the virus spread, many facilities faced staff shortages due to employees being exposed to or becoming sick with the disease. Some facilities couldn't isolate infected residents properly (or at all), contributing to rapid spread of the virus.

Many facilities also had extremely inadequate communication with the families of their residents. In some cases, facilities didn't promptly inform families when their loved ones became ill or even after they died, and the public was furious about the lack of transparency and accountability. Many families tried to get their loved ones out of assisted-living facilities, especially if they received news of a positive case in the facility where they lived.

According to a report by the Kaiser Family Foundation, as of April 2021, U.S. long-term care facility residents and staff accounted for 8 percent of the cases of COVID-19 but a staggering 32 percent of the deaths from COVID-19. This tragedy underscored the need for substantial changes (primarily at the state and local levels) to protect residents of these facilities.

Innovating to Counteract Pandemic Challenges

One of the shiniest silver linings of the pandemic involves how many innovative solutions people found to overcome the problems at hand. So many innovations arose that I can't possibly include all of them here (that topic could be at least one book on its own). But I highlight a few of these groundbreaking ideas in the following sections.

In the medical field

Obviously, some of the biggest innovations of the COVID-19 pandemic related to the efforts of the medical industry to deal with the virus. These big ideas include

» **COVID-19 treatments and vaccines:** Out of necessity, researchers developed treatments (see Chapter 8) and vaccines (see Chapter 6) at record speeds. These responses to the pandemic provide some of the most important healthcare innovations of the decade.

» **Tracking mechanisms for pandemic-related information:** Scientists used artificial intelligence (AI) in unprecedented ways to perform contact tracing, infection prediction modeling, and patient care. For example, some companies provided doctors with AI tools to help them make correct diagnoses and specific treatment plans remotely, based on symptoms and telehealth interviews.

» **3D printing technology:** Many people across different fields pitched in to fast-track the design and printing of medical equipment — including masks, face shields, and respiratory care equipment — that supported efforts to combat the pandemic.

» **Telehealth services:** Medical staff expanded the use of these services exponentially, giving patients remote access to medical professionals they couldn't otherwise reach for consultation, treatment, and mental health support.

In other industries

Other industries have made innovative changes to how and where they operate, as well as the tools that they use. Some examples include

>> **Enhanced online learning:** In education, developers enhanced online learning platforms to make them more interactive and user-friendly. For example, they incorporated innovative approaches such as *flipped classrooms* (where students complete homework during class time and view lectures on their own time) and *personalized learning* (which aims to target the learning experience to individual student's strengths, needs, interests, and so on).

Moreover, educators have become more adept at leveraging technology to reach and engage students effectively, reshaping the educational landscape for the post-pandemic world.

>> **Business operations and services:** In the corporate world, businesses have rapidly adapted to new ways of working, including developing more sophisticated and shareable digital collaboration tools, project management software, and cloud services. Companies have created ways to provide contactless services, digital transactions, and virtual consultations.

>> **Advances in automation and virtual reality platforms:** The pandemic accelerated the automation trend, leading to a surge in the use of robotics and AI in industries such as manufacturing (training AI to recognize and remove defects during quality control), logistics (using robots to find and pick items in warehouses), retail (increasing contactless/cashierless checkout), and entertainment (expanding virtual video games and universes). Also, people flocked to virtual socialization platforms, from online gaming communities to digital concerts.

During the pandemic, developers used augmented and virtual reality technologies to create immersive experiences for isolated individuals and provide a way to escape during lockdowns. Most of these developments — including the Facebook Metaverse — are still in full swing today.

>> **Remote auditions:** As for the world of acting, during the pandemic, nobody could audition in person, so the casting agencies started accepting self-tapes, which became the preferred audition method. Self-taping has opened up more roles to more people in locations around the world.

In the end, the pandemic was truly awful, but the world can't deny that many people and companies expertly pivoted during the pandemic to create something entirely new for their customers, clients, and the world at large. The innovation that happened during the pandemic was unique, and it's still going on.

Working and Schooling Remotely

One of the most wide-reaching results of the pandemic across the globe was the advent of mainstream remote work and remote schooling.

Embracing the virtual workplace

Although remote working wasn't a new concept before COVID-19 hit, the pandemic did push employers into a corner, and they had to accept employees working remotely as the only option if they wanted to stay in business. Many companies are still operating remotely (partially or fully) today, taking advantage of benefits such as

>> **Flexibility:** Employees can work from anywhere, eliminating commute times and giving them a greater ability to balance work and life. Trusting employees with their own schedules also improves morale and employee satisfaction.

>> **Productivity:** Many companies have seen their workforce become more efficient and productive because they can work without office interruptions.

>> **Cost-savings:** Companies have reduced what they spend on renting physical office space, buying office supplies, and paying for office utilities; employees can save on commuting, meal costs, and work clothes.

Just like anything else, remote working has potential pitfalls and downsides, too. For example

>> **No boundaries:** The lack of separation between work and personal life can backfire and lead to bosses expecting employees to work at any hour around the clock.

>> **Limited team building:** Virtual teams might struggle with building strong interpersonal relationships, which could affect team cohesion and morale.

>> **Technical access:** Not everyone has a reliable Internet connection, current equipment, or a suitable working environment at home (or in the cafe down the street, after the pandemic lockdowns lifted).

Adapting to remote education

At the time that the COVID-19 pandemic started, remote schooling was a new concept to many school districts and students around the world. When the pandemic hit, most schools didn't have the infrastructure, precedent, or policies in place to successfully put all of their students online immediately, and students and teachers alike faced many challenges, such as

>> **The Digital Divide:** Many students don't have access to reliable electricity, let alone to an Internet connection. They also may not have computers, tablets, or other equipment for online learning, leading to disparities in education quality caused by this lack of resources.

>> **Distracting, embarrassing, or unstable home life:** Some children live in homes that are too hectic for them to concentrate on schoolwork, that embarrass the students in some way, or that are actually unsafe for them to be there, and they therefore cannot concentrate on school. It's impossible for a child to concentrate on schooling if they're worried about being verbally or physically abused.

>> **Food insecurity:** Many children qualify for free breakfasts and lunches through various U.S. school programs, and although most school districts continued their programs via pickup or drive-throughs, some students still couldn't access these vital meals.

>> **Lost quality socializing:** Without recess, lunch, and other non-structured time between classes, students really missed out on having friends and social time face to face. Many children felt isolated, depressed, and anxious without these lost connections.

Today, many students (especially if they were very young during the pandemic) struggle with social anxiety and basic interactions that they never had the opportunity to become familiar with at the optimal point in their development.

>> **Increased screen time:** Students as young as kindergarten had to sit in front of screens for six or more hours per day, which can cause health issues even in adults. Especially for kids, extensive screen exposure can lead to eye strain and vision problems, headaches, and sleeping problems.

On the other hand, remote learning was really the best hand everyone could play with the cards that the pandemic dealt them. And the move to remote classrooms wasn't all bad; it had some benefits, including

>> **Increased safety from infection:** Remote learning eliminates the risk of disease transmission among students and teachers.

>> **Getting access to digital resources:** Which can make learning more interactive and engaging for some students.

>> **Developing digital literacy:** Whether they were beginners or proficient before the pandemic, students attending remote schooling improved their technical skills by using digital technologies to connect with their teachers and classrooms. This knowledge helps prepare them for the increasingly digital world they live in.

Overall, some students did really well (or even better) when schooling went remote. Others struggled greatly. But at least all students now know remote learning is an option, which may open up a world of possibilities for them if they don't feel safe or productive in traditional schools.

CHALLENGES FOR THE REMOTE TEACHERS

From the educators' standpoint, some teachers really liked engaging a remote classroom and have gone on to teach only remote classes. Others very much struggled to teach classes while caring for and supervising the education of their own children, who were also participating in remote learning from their bedrooms.

According to the paper "Teacher Burnout in the Time of COVID-19: Antecedents and Psychological Consequences" (published in the February 27, 2023, issue of *International Journal of Environmental Research and Public Health:* www.ncbi.nlm.nih.gov/pmc/articles/PMC10002371/), many teachers felt burnt out and inadequately prepared and supported to successfully manage and teach remotely. And that situation became more challenging after schools opened up again. After reopening, many schools offered a *hybrid model* at first, where teachers interacted with some students in the classroom while others watched via live video stream.

Many teachers found that the hybrid model didn't allow them to give full attention to any students. If the teacher taught to the in-classroom students, the online students got neglected, and vice versa. Teaching (and learning) in that way took quite a toll on everyone.

A Look at Healthcare System Impacts

The COVID-19 pandemic placed an extraordinary burden on healthcare systems worldwide, leading to a reduction in preventative medical treatment, as well as healthcare system overloads and healthcare worker burnout.

Reduced preventative healthcare

During the pandemic, preventative healthcare decreased to almost none at all. Most of our healthcare workers had to use their limited work hours to help manage the crisis. In turn, all non-essential or routine health services were delayed or suspended altogether for many months, if not a year or more. No annual exams. No teeth cleanings. No Pap smears or mammograms. No elective surgeries. If someone were in immediate danger of dying, they could get medical assistance. But missing basic services certainly meant that some people might miss early detection and prevention of potential deadly conditions. Consider these situations:

>> People living with conditions such as hypertension, diabetes, and cardiovascular diseases may have experienced worsening in their conditions and couldn't receive the proper timely treatment, putting them at risk of complications and even death.

>> Even if they could find preventative treatment, many people didn't want to go to the doctor or hospital anyway because they didn't want to catch COVID-19 in that environment.

>> Equally troubling, people seemed to have a reluctance to seek mental health services. Failure to diagnose and treat emotional needs can lead to more severe health (emotional and physical) outcomes down the line.

Overload and worker burnout

While the hospitals flooded with COVID-19 patients beyond capacity, the pressure on healthcare facilities and many of the world's medical systems may never fully recover from the failure of the infrastructure and the impact on healthcare workers. So how did this failure happen? Here are some reasons why COVID-19 nearly caused the collapse of the healthcare system:

>> The number of patients requiring intensive, around-the-clock care constantly increased, and it did so exponentially. At the height of the pandemic, improvised temporary facilities to house and care for these patients took the form of hallways, conference rooms, and even outdoor tents.

>> Hospitals didn't have enough personal protective equipment (PPE), such as masks and respirators; ventilators for the patients who had severe respiratory distress; or even hospital beds.

>> Hospitals had to still treat non-COVID patients, on top of COVID-19 patients, while keeping the two populations separated. This separation was often difficult — or impossible — to accomplish in overcrowded emergency departments, especially before widespread testing was available.

In addition to these factors, we all, as healthcare workers, also faced

>> **Outrageously demanding work schedules and chronic stress:** A high patient load and low staffing — when employees got sick or left the healthcare workforce entirely — led to physical and mental exhaustion.

>> **Working in extremely risky conditions:** Some healthcare workers didn't have proper PPE, and they worried that they would contract COVID-19 and pass it on to their families.

Many workers went through extensive disinfection procedures every time they came home. Some *didn't even go home*, especially if they had young, old, or sick family members at home.

>> **Witnessing high rates of morbidity and mortality every day:** Having healthcare workers exposed to constant loss without having time to process it created deep trauma, leading to nightmares, dissociation, and other disorders and coping behaviors that require mental health care.

Even though some workers received mental health support and interventions, some may have needed more. Many healthcare workers worked under extreme duress, while physically sick in some cases themselves. And some watched their coworkers die.

>> **Making high-stake decisions under immense pressure:** At times, the hands-on healthcare workers had to make hard decisions about which patients would receive immediate attention. They also needed to decide on treatment and isolation before there was adequate information to support these decisions.

To this day, the impact on healthcare workers may be severe and permanent. Burnout remains a critical issue, and facilities have seen a massive reduction in staffing because of healthcare workers leaving their professions since the pandemic.

The pandemic put a huge spotlight on how inadequate and vulnerable the world's healthcare systems truly are. Governments, public healthcare officials, and hospital administrators must work together to strengthen their healthcare systems and provide comprehensive support for healthcare workers. Prior to the pandemic, hospital leadership in many countries reduced healthcare costs by reducing hospital bed numbers. However, the COVID-19 pandemic demonstrated that hospitals need to be able to rapidly increase the number of available hospital beds in case of an emergency (known as *surge capacity*), and hospitals worldwide must make changes to improve their surge capacities.

Increased Intergenerational Living

For better or worse, the pandemic prompted a resurgence in intergenerational living that the U.S. hasn't seen for decades. Although it peaked during the pandemic, many families have maintained this living arrangement, for many reasons:

>> **Different generations can support each other physically and emotionally.** Older adults can share their wisdom and experience, while younger ones can assist with physical tasks and technology.

>> **Sharing a household saves money.** For example, you have one mortgage or rent payment per month, rather than two (or more).

>> **Families living together can share and preserve cultural traditions.** These traditions include recipes, history, and language.

>> **Living together with family members prevents isolation.** Although it's particularly a concern for older people, younger people can have just as much of a problem with isolation.

Now, intergenerational living isn't all sunshine and roses, and it doesn't work for everyone. Some potential drawbacks to consider are

>> **Potential conflicts:** Differences in values, parenting styles, and lifestyle preferences can lead to conflicts.

>> **Increased care demands:** Caring for elderly relatives can add stress and burden to working adults, potentially leading to caregiver burnout. And if you have young kids in the mix, the caregivers become what's called the *sandwich generation,* having to care for people on both ends of the age spectrum, which is especially exhausting.

>> **Risks for disease transmission:** An increased risk of transmitting COVID-19 (or other illnesses) to vulnerable older adults. And if small kids (who are normally germ factories) live in the same house, trying to prevent shared infections can get gnarly pretty quickly.

TIP

Although living with multiple generations in one household offers many benefits, it also brings challenges. If you decide to try it with your family, make sure to establish boundaries, promote open communication, and give each other a lot of patience, grace, and trust.

Supply Chain Disruptions, Hoarding, and Shortages

Some of the more specific markers of the COVID-19 pandemic were supply chain disruptions, supply shortages, and hoarding.

When the reality of the pandemic hit, consumers around the world started hoarding essential items out of fear of future shortages and lockdowns. People bought up supplies in quantities that far exceeded the regular consumption rates. How could anyone forget that people hoarded toilet paper, hand sanitizer, and cleaning supplies? For food items, people especially stocked up on staples such as pasta, rice, and canned goods.

And at the same time, supply chain disruptions reduced the availability of fresh produce, meat, and dairy products. Here are other examples of shortages:

>> **In the healthcare sector,** the demand for personal protective equipment (PPE) — such as masks, gloves, and gowns — far outstripped the supply, causing shortages. Some healthcare workers didn't have enough equipment and gear to protect themselves from getting sick.

>> **Retailers** didn't have the supply of their regular goods because lockdowns and other public health and safety measures slowed down or halted production in many industries. Plus, travel restrictions and reduced staffing created delays and disruptions in delivering goods from manufacturers to retailers.

>> **The automotive industry** experienced a significant shortage of semiconductors, an essential component in modern vehicles. Many semiconductor factories had to shut down or reduce their production due to the pandemic. And at the same time, the demand for semiconductors surged because of an increase in electronics sales when people started working (and going to school) from home. This semiconductor demand led to a severe shortage that affected automotive production worldwide just as the demand for automobiles in many urban areas increased due to fear of using mass transportation.

2

Staying Safe and Healthy

Uncover everything you need to know about how COVID-19 is transmitted.

Prevent and mitigate the spread of COVID-19.

Find out whether you have COVID-19.

Receive care for mild to severe COVID-19.

Live life with Long COVID.

Chapter **5**

Transmitting COVID-19

A t the time of writing, the world has been living with COVID-19 for several years, and the medical community knows a good amount about how people spread it — and therefore, how to prevent it. Effective prevention measures benefit the overall health and wellness of the world's population, as long as people stay current on recent developments and use good hygiene practices.

In this chapter, I walk you through exactly how SARS-CoV-2, the virus that causes COVID-19, spreads among people. I dispel common myths about transmission, give you tips and pointers about how to stay COVID-negative, and help you figure out how contagious you are when you do test positive.

Exploring How COVID-19 Is Transmitted

COVID-19 spreads when someone who's infected with the SARS-CoV-2 virus coughs, sneezes, or otherwise releases particles of fluid into the air, and then someone else comes into contact with that fluid. The virus can also live on surfaces, which means that if you touch a surface contaminated by particles containing the virus, you can potentially become infected — although people don't commonly transmit the virus in this way.

You can catch COVID-19 in three main ways:

>> Having contaminated particles come in contact with your mouth, eyes, or nose

>> Breathing in air that contains contaminated particles

>> Getting contaminated particles from the air or surfaces onto your hands, and then touching your eyes, nose, or mouth with your hands (the least likely way to catch COVID-19)

REMEMBER

You're most at risk of contracting COVID-19 from an infected person if you're within 6 feet of them, and either or both of you are unmasked. Find out more about masking in Chapter 6 and in the section "Knowing the nature of droplets and aerosols," later in this chapter.

Exploring droplet versus airborne transmission

COVID-19 primarily spreads through fairly large liquid particles known as *droplets*, which are tiny bits of mucus and/or saliva that exit your mouth and nose when you cough, sneeze, or even sing or speak.

These large droplets are visible to the naked eye and relatively heavy, which is why you can often feel them hit you. Due to their weight, they can only travel through the air for at most 6 feet before they fall onto whatever surfaces lie beneath, whether that's furniture (such as a table) or the ground.

If another person is within 6 feet of those droplets, the droplets may land on the person, rather than a surface. The closer you are to an infected person, the more likely you are to come into contact with any droplets they emit — and if the droplets land in your mouth, eyes, or nose, then you may contract COVID-19.

Knowing the nature of droplets and aerosols

Although droplet transmission as a regular topic of conversation didn't become a mainstream habit until the pandemic, droplets themselves aren't new. For as long as people have existed (really, even before people existed), droplets have been flying through the air. Everyone has been spat on inadvertently by someone else (and everyone has probably done the spitting at some point).

You (and those around you) can find spreading droplets by expelling them from your mouth or nose annoying and embarrassing, but this droplet spread can also create a health hazard because a lot of different viruses and bacteria can transmit through droplets. The old saying, "Say it, don't spray it," isn't just a cute insult. It reminds us all to practice good health consciousness, especially in a post-COVID world.

If you maintain a distance of 6 feet or greater from an infected person, you have a much lower chance of encountering any droplets that they produce and expel. And if you add on a mask (to one or both of you), the chances of contracting this (or other) viruses or bacteria decrease even further. (You can find more details about the ins and outs of masking in Chapter 6.)

In addition to droplets, you can also contract COVID-19 through smaller microdroplets known as *aerosol particles.* The general term *aerosols* describes any very small particles — liquid or solid — that travel suspended in the air. Aerosols are much lighter than droplets. You can spread aerosol particles through normal breathing and talking.

For example, if you're COVID-positive, you can emit aerosol particles into the air while simply taking a regular chat break around the office water cooler, and others can easily breathe in that aerosol. After the aerosol particles enter someone else's lungs, the virus can settle in.

Emitting aerosol particles is one of the ways in which asymptomatic, COVID-positive people spread COVID. See Chapter 11 for more information about this type of spreading.

Avoiding the scourge of airborne transmission

When doctors talk about *airborne transmission,* we mean aerosol transmission (discussed in the preceding section). Even though larger droplets travel through the air for a little while, experts in infection control don't consider them airborne because they fall quickly to the ground. On the other hand, aerosols stay suspended in the air itself.

Because they weigh so little, aerosols stay suspended in the air for up to a half hour, depending on the environment. If you're outside in a nice open area that has a good breeze, aerosols disperse quickly. If you're indoors or you don't have good air circulation in an outdoor setting (think of being on a semi-enclosed porch on a hot, humid day), then the aerosol doesn't disperse as quickly.

Even though aerosol transmission is typically less common for COVID-19, you can still catch COVID-19 from aerosol particles because of how long they remain in the air, and how easily and quickly you can breathe in large numbers of the particles without even realizing it.

Although the biggest culprit of COVID-19 transmission involves contracting droplets at close range, you can also get and give COVID-19 through airborne/aerosol transmission. You have a greater likelihood of contracting COVID from aerosols when you're

>> **Indoors with a lot of people for an extended period of time:** The close proximity and reduced air movement mean you have a greater chance of encountering the virus than you would outdoors.

>> **Unmasked and close to someone who's expelling a large number of viruses:** For example, someone near you might be coughing or sneezing.

>> **Engaged in activities such as singing or shouting:** Because those activities expel a lot of droplets and aerosols into the air.

>> **You're in a poorly ventilated area:** A lack of air movement means no way to clear out aerosols.

TIP

When you host or attend large indoor gatherings, ensure that your location has proper ventilation and circulation of fresh air. To read more about how you can prevent the spread of COVID-19, flip to Chapter 6.

Surfaces: Not as scary as we thought

Although many viruses and bacteria leave no trace after a drop-let (or microdroplet) that contains them lands on a surface and evaporates, some germs remain after the droplet is gone, and those can infect you. The COVID-19 virus falls into the latter cat-egory. When surfaces have infectious particles on them, the sur-faces are known as *fomites.* If you touch a fomite and then touch your mouth, nose, or eyes, you may transfer virus particles (or bacteria) into your body.

Consider this: If someone coughs or sneezes in front of you, your brain zeroes right in on that, and you can respond immediately to protect yourself. For example, you can move a few steps away, excuse yourself altogether, or wash your hands.

But if you absentmindedly touch the surface of a table during a meeting, you don't usually consciously think of the germs that you might pick up. But if someone who's infected with the SARS-CoV-2 virus turned that table into a fomite, your contact with that fomite exposes you to the virus. If you go on about your day without washing your hands after that meeting and at some point, touch your eyes, nose, or mouth, you risk contracting COVID-19. That's the bad news.

REMEMBER

I have good news, too: Surface transmission of COVID-19 isn't the big bad scary beast that we used to think it was. Although you technically can catch COVID-19 from a surface, fomite transmission is much less likely than person-to-person transmission. In the beginning of the pandemic, the medical community thought that people might spread COVID-19 on surfaces just as quickly and easily as they could through droplet transmission. But studies of acquisition of COVID-19 indicate that fomite transmission happens much less frequently than transmission through the air.

SUPERSPREADER EVENTS

Because droplet transmission is the most potent way to spread COVID-19, when you get a lot of people together in very close quarters, COVID-19 can spread very far, very quickly. One infected person can contaminate multiple people with one sneeze or cough.

Early in the pandemic, large, unmasked group gatherings led to big numbers of COVID-19 cases, stretching far beyond the original gathering's attendees. The attendees who contracted COVID-19 without knowing it just went about their lives. In the course of their normal routine, they spread the virus to others who didn't even attend the gathering. Experts in infection control call these incidents *superspreader events.*

Of course, not every single large gathering becomes a superspreader event. Scientists don't quite know why yet. But they do know how just

(continued)

(continued)

a few people can cause a superspreader event. Using a model based on real world data, researchers found and reported (in the May 2022 issue of the journal *Physics of Fluids*) that about 80 percent of infections at superspreader events came from only 4 percent of all contagious attendees. One explanation suggests that the COVID-positive people who had higher viral loads spread the virus more easily and quickly because of the density of virus in the droplets that they expelled. Also, gatherings have great potential to become superspreader events if they're indoors without proper ventilation and people don't wear masks while singing or shouting.

Now that more people have received COVID-19 vaccinations, everyone knows more about ventilation in relation to reducing risk, and some people still use masks, large gatherings typically aren't the big spreaders they used to be.

Sorting Through Symptoms

Even before COVID-19 came on the scene, people asked themselves these questions when they experienced certain symptoms:

>> Is this a cold or the flu — or just allergies?

>> Is this a stomach virus or food poisoning?

>> Should I go to the doctor or just ride this thing out?

Now that COVID-19 has appeared on the scene, you may struggle with making sense of what's producing symptoms of illness and what kind of care you should get when you feel sick.

COVID-19 has wide and varied symptoms, and those symptoms overlap with symptoms of other illnesses. On top of that, some people can have very mild or barely noticeable symptoms, while others experience major illness — which can even sometimes stretch on for months or years. (For more on Long COVID, turn to Chapter 9.) Common symptoms of COVID-19 include

>> Fever or chills

>> Cough

>> Shortness of breath

- » Fatigue
- » Muscle or body aches
- » Headache
- » New loss of taste or smell
- » Sore throat
- » Congestion or runny nose
- » Nausea or vomiting
- » Diarrhea

The preceding list includes only symptoms that the medical community knows so far. With each variant, new symptoms emerge. For example, in early 2023, the Centers for Disease Control and Prevention (CDC) warned that *conjunctivitis* (pink eye) can also be a symptom of certain strains of COVID-19.

You might look at the preceding list and think, "Gosh, a lot of these symptoms are also flu symptoms. How can I tell the difference?" So glad you asked; I help you figure out what illness your symptoms indicate in the following sections.

WARNING

Some symptoms of COVID-19 are extremely serious. Call your local EMS or get to an emergency room immediately if you or someone you know has

- » Trouble breathing
- » Persistent pain or pressure in the chest
- » New confusion
- » Inability to wake or stay awake
- » Pale, gray, or blue-colored skin, lips, or nail beds (depending on your skin tone)

Differentiating COVID-19, the Flu, and a Cold

Colds, allergies, the flu, or COVID-19 — how the heck do you know what you have? You can start by evaluating the most obvious distinguishing symptoms.

When a cold is the suspect

If you have a cold, your symptoms may include

>> Runny nose

>> Cough

>> Congestion

>> Sore throat

TIP

You know that you have a cold, and not the flu or COVID-19, if you have pretty mild symptoms from the preceding list, and you don't have aches or a fever. If you can still function (with or without over-the-counter cold medicine), and you feel all better in just a few days, you probably have a regular case of the sniffles — hooray!

But if you have a fever or feel a bit achy, you probably have more than a cold. The following section discusses figuring out whether you have the flu or COVID-19.

The flu versus COVID-19

Because the flu and COVID-19 are both highly contagious respiratory illnesses, they do present very similarly, and you really may not know for sure which one you have without taking a test. You can even ask your doctor for a combo flu/COVID-19 test (more on testing in Chapter 7).

Nonetheless, a few anecdotal differences may help clue you in:

>> **Onset:** The onset of COVID-19 is gradual, but the flu usually strikes rapidly.

>> **Length of illness:** Whereas flu symptoms tend to last anywhere from one to about four days (at the *very* outside, two weeks), COVID-19 symptoms can last up to two weeks — or even longer.

>> **Severity:** Although not always the case, COVID-19 may make you sicker than the flu. By *sicker*, I mean: You can feel worse, have more severe symptoms, and may be ill for longer.

>> **Complications:** COVID-19 (and sometimes the flu) can cause severe complications that require you to go to the hospital. (See the following section for those complications.)

Complications from either one

Some of the complications from either the flu or COVID-19 include

>> *Pneumonia* (infection in the lungs)

>> Respiratory failure

>> *Pulmonary edema* (fluid in the lungs)

>> *Sepsis* (life-threatening inflammation throughout the body)

>> Strokes or heart attacks

>> *Pulmonary emboli* (blood clots in the lungs)

>> Worsening of chronic medical conditions (especially diabetes or conditions involving the lungs, heart, or nervous system)

>> Inflammation of the heart, brain, or muscles

>> Secondary infections

REMEMBER

COVID-19 and the flu share the preceding list of potential complications, but COVID-19 especially comes with the risk of blood clots.

Got all that? Although you may find keeping track of the differences difficult, if you look at the symptoms and how prevalent they are side-by-side in Table 5-1, you may find it a bit easier to navigate. This table shows only the symptoms that differ between the flu and COVID-19.

TABLE 5-1 ## Differences in Symptoms

Symptom	Flu	COVID-19
Onset	Rapid	Gradual
Shortness of breath	Rare	Common
Fatigue	Often	Occasionally
Loss of taste	Rarely	Occasionally
Sneezing	Rarely	No

Knowing When and for How Long You're Contagious

All viruses have a specific *incubation period*, which is how many days it takes for you to see symptoms after you become infected.

Different COVID-19 variants have different incubation periods, but on average, most people contract COVID-19 and show symptoms about 5 or 6 days after exposure — although symptoms can emerge as early as 2 days after exposure and as late as 12 days. The Omicron variant seems to have a shorter incubation period than the original COVID-19 strain, at around 3 days. And it doesn't happen often, but you can first show symptoms as long as 14 days after infection.

When you become contagious

After you become infected with COVID-19, you can spread the virus for 48 hours before your symptoms begin, and you're most contagious throughout the first five days after your symptoms start. You become less infectious after day 5, but technically, you can still spread the virus beyond the first five days.

If you remain asymptomatic but test positive for COVID-19, you're still most infectious in the five days after your exposure.

How long you're contagious

Everyone has a different immune response to a virus, so everyone remains contagious for different lengths of time. Most people are no longer infectious after day 10 (especially if they have a mild case and their symptoms improve in a few days with resolution of fever). However, if you have a severe case of COVID-19 or have a weakened immune system, you can remain contagious for as long as 30 days after the start of your symptoms.

Get vaccinated! If you're vaccinated and become infected with COVID-19, you very well may never become contagious. And if you are contagious at all, you probably won't stay contagious for as long as depicted in Figure 5-1. (The figure is based on information from the article "How Long Are You Contagious with COVID-19," written by Ronald W. Dworkin, MD, PhD and reviewed by Patricia Pinto-Garcia, MD, MPH; GoodRxHealth, October 12, 2022). Also, people who take antiviral medications are much less likely to be contagious. I go over vaccines in more detail in Chapter 6, and cover more about antivirals in Chapter 8.

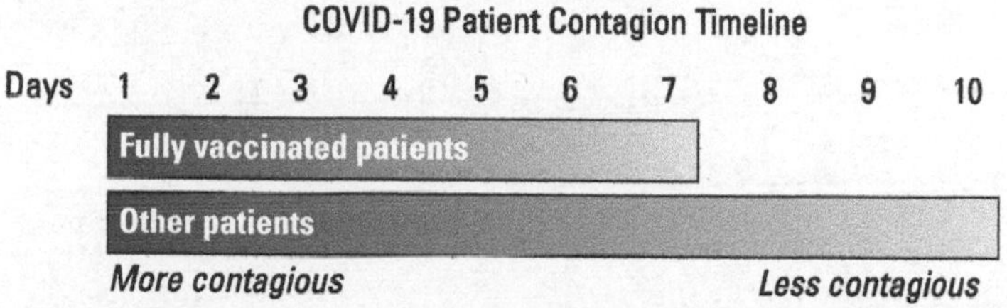

COVID-19 Patient Contagion Timeline

Days	1	2	3	4	5	6	7	8	9	10

Fully vaccinated patients

Other patients

More contagious   *Less contagious*

FIGURE 5-1: The COVID-19 vaccine helps shorten the time period that you're contagious.

IN THIS CHAPTER

» **Using mRNA vaccines to prevent illness**

» **Getting all the details about getting vaccinated**

» **Mastering masking**

» **Weighing the risks of indoor and outdoor gatherings**

» **Highlighting habits to stay healthy**

Chapter **6**

Protecting Yourself and Others from COVID-19

The world now has COVID-19 under control because people figured out how to avoid spreading it and committed to healthy and hygienic practices. Many government and public health agencies created laws and mandates requiring the public to follow the best practices and guidelines that medical professionals devised to combat the spread of COVID-19.

Although the pandemic that began in 2020 is in the past, continuing practices such as receiving regular vaccinations, masking when you are sick or exposed to someone who is sick, and quarantining and isolating (as needed) can keep us all safer from the virus (as well as other illnesses).

In this chapter, I explain how mRNA vaccine technology revolutionized the way in which people can protect themselves and what you can expect when you get your COVID-19 vaccine. I also go over why continuing the practice of masking can still make a difference and describe other healthy habits that you can adopt to keep your immune system in tip-top shape and ready to fight COVID-19 and other infections.

Tackling COVID-19 with mRNA Vaccines

Of the three different types of COVID-19 vaccines (mRNA, protein subunit, and viral vector), researchers generally consider the mRNA vaccines the most significant scientific breakthrough of the pandemic. I cover the basics of all three types in Chapter 2 (in case you need that coverage), but in this chapter, I add a little more detail to explain how mRNA vaccine technology provided such a breakthrough for the COVID-19 pandemic and beyond.

Instead of using components of the COVID-19 virus to teach your body how to respond to the illness (which the other two vaccine types do), mRNA vaccines use a lab-generated genetic code that triggers your body to make proteins that train your immune system. This method gives scientists a way to easily replicate the vaccine-creation process for many other infections by inserting the genetic code for other germs into the same vaccine backbone.

Thanks to the work of researchers around the world — foremost among them, Penn Medicine/University of Pennsylvania's Katalin Kariko, Ph.D., and Drew Weissman, M.D., Ph.D. — scientists were already developing mRNA vaccine technology well before COVID-19 arrived. So when the pandemic hit, the researchers were ready to put the mRNA technology into action.

Many governments around the world tracked and reported the number of COVID-19 vaccines that their citizens received during the pandemic, but global tracking stopped after the CDC declared that the pandemic became contained in May 2023. Nonetheless, the tracking shows that people around the world have received more than 10 billion doses of the vaccine, which has proven safe and effective.

REMEMBER

The original mRNA vaccine was *monovalent,* which means that it offered protection against just one strain of the virus. As of August 2022, all COVID-19 vaccines became *bivalent,* which means they contain mRNA genetic codes from two strains of the virus — the original strain and an Omicron variant. This bivalent vaccine provides better protection against the virus, even if you already became infected with and recovered from COVID-19.

Getting Vaccinated

Getting vaccinated offers your greatest weapon against COVID-19. Even though getting the vaccine doesn't guarantee that you'll never get COVID-19, it does significantly reduce your chances of getting sick when you come into contact with the virus. Also, if you do get COVID-19 after receiving a vaccination, you're much less likely to

>> Become extremely sick

>> Need hospitalization

>> Contract Long COVID

>> Die from COVID-19 complications

Knowing what to expect

You receive the COVID-19 vaccine like many other vaccines: in the form of an injection. You can find the vaccines available in many places, such as

>> **Your doctor's office:** You may need an appointment.

>> **Pop-up clinics or urgent care facilities:** You can often walk into these without an appointment.

>> **Many drugstores and pharmacies:** You can schedule an appointment on the store's website or by calling them. In most cases, COVID-19 vaccines are free to patients through insurance, Medicare, Medicaid, or other government funding.

>> **Your own home:** If you're homebound, you have several ways you can schedule a visit from a medical provider who can vaccinate you in your home:

- Call your healthcare provider
- Visit your county or state's health department website
- Contact the Aging Network online or via telephone (800-677-1116)
- Search for services by ZIP code on the Eldercare Locator (https://eldercare.acl.gov/Public/Index.aspx)
- Call the Disability Information and Access Line (888-677-1199)
- Call the Medicare hotline (800-633-4227)

Regardless of the location where you decide to receive your shot, getting the COVID-19 vaccine is pretty straightforward. You usually follow some version of these steps:

1. **Fill out any paperwork that the location you chose requires, such as a pre-vaccination checklist.**

   This checklist asks you questions such as whether you have symptoms, believe you've been in contact with an infected person, and what your basic medical history is.

2. **Tell the medical provider in which arm you want to receive the shot.**

   The provider then cleans a small spot on your chosen upper arm by using an alcohol pad.

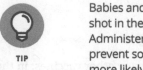

TIP

   Babies and children who have small arm muscles may get the shot in their thigh, where they have a larger muscle. Administering the vaccine in a larger muscle can help to prevent soreness and adverse reactions. Also, the vaccine is more likely to be completely injected within that larger muscle, which increases its effectiveness.

3. **Relax as much as possible while you receive the shot because if the muscle is relaxed, the shot won't hurt as much.**

   The provider then covers the shot spot with a bandage, or a cotton ball or gauze pad covered with medical tape.

4. **Take a seat in the designated observation area for about 15 minutes.**

   During the period of observation, the provider monitors you for any signs of adverse reactions to the vaccine, such as difficulty breathing, dizziness, or chest pain.

5. **After the 15 minutes elapse (and you have no adverse reactions), feel free to go about your business.**

   Or just go home and take care of yourself!

Dealing with soreness or other side effects

The COVID-19 shot goes right into your muscle. While the liquid goes in, it slightly stretches your muscle, which can create soreness later. All muscles have this normal response to getting overused or inflamed, and the soreness should resolve itself in a few days.

If you're worried that you won't be able to use your arm normally for a couple of days, choose your non-dominant arm for the shot.

To keep pain and potential soreness at bay, remember these tips when getting your COVID-19 vaccine:

>> **Move your arm** afterwards to promote blood flow. Here are two easy ways:

- Stretch your arm across your chest.
- Let your arm dangle in its natural position at your side. Then, lift your arm straight out to the side until you get to shoulder level.

  Do three sets of ten repetitions a few times throughout the day after your shot to make sure you continue to promote blood flow to the arm.

>> **Place an ice pack or cold compress on your arm** for up to 15 minutes at a time throughout the day if you develop soreness at the vaccine site. If cold doesn't help, you can try a warm compress, instead.

>> **Take an analgesic medication,** such as acetaminophen or ibuprofen, afterwards to help limit the inflammation and pain.

  Don't take an analgesic before you get your vaccine shot because scientists haven't studied the use of painkillers enough to know how much they may affect your immune system. Although they don't know for sure, there is a chance that analgesics can weaken your immune system, and taking them before you get a vaccine may decrease its effectiveness.

>> **Take it easy!** Try to get your shot on a day in which you don't need to do much, if possible.

In addition to arm soreness, you may experience other common side effects — *don't worry* if you experience any of these symptoms:

>> Swelling or redness on your arm
>> Fever
>> Chills
>> Nausea
>> Headache
>> Fatigue

Children may have slightly different side effects, such as

>> Crying and feeling irritable
>> Swollen lymph nodes
>> No appetite

REMEMBER

These side-effect symptoms won't harm you, and in fact, they indicate that the vaccine is working — it's causing your immune system to respond to it. Getting the vaccine affects everyone differently. Some people have no symptoms at all, some just feel tired and sleepy for a day or two, and still others feel super sick.

In general, expect to feel like your normal self again within one or two days. You can try to mitigate the impact that the vaccine tiredness may have on your daily life:

>> Schedule your vaccine appointment for a time when you can rest and take care of yourself as much as you need without worrying about working or household duties.

>> Get some help from family or friends if you need childcare or other responsibilities covered while you rest.

>> Definitely don't schedule your vaccine injection to happen right before anything that you can't cancel if you have to.

WARNING

Although it's extremely rare, you can potentially experience unexpected adverse or allergic reactions to the vaccine. These types of reactions appear as late as six weeks after you receive the shot. If you experience any severe reaction, call 911 or get to an emergency room immediately. Some known adverse reactions include

>> **Anaphylaxis:** An immediate severe allergic reaction that results in symptoms such as a racing heart, shortness of breath or wheezing, lightheadedness, or collapsing.

>> **Myocarditis or pericarditis:** A condition in which your heart (*myocardium*) or heart lining (*pericardium*) becomes inflamed. You may experience symptoms such as a racing heart, chest pain, or shortness of breath. This heart inflammation occurs rarely in adolescents who receive the COVID-19 vaccine, and almost always goes away in a few days without any further effects.

Following up with your vaccine provider

Your medical provider, the CDC, or the local health department may ask — when you sign up for your appointment, during your appointment, or after your appointment — if you want to opt-in to receive text messages that check in on your recovery. If you opt to receive these messages, you receive automatic messages that ask you how you're feeling and request a description of any symptoms that you may have. Receiving follow-up messaging allows you to share data that can help improve the COVID-19 vaccine and also access guidance if you do experience symptoms.

Additionally, you need to revisit your vaccine provider to receive a one, two-, or three-shot series in order for the vaccine manufacturer, the USFDA, and the WHO to consider you fully vaccinated (which means you've received all doses of the vaccine as outlined by the FDA, WHO, and manufacturer). All vaccine types are equally effective, so you get to decide whether you get a vaccine that mandates just one or multiple doses based on your personal preference and what's available near you.

Determining Who Should Get Vaccinated

The CDC recommends that all people ages 6 months and older get vaccinated against COVID-19. Children and babies receive the same vaccine that adults do, just in a smaller dose.

WARNING

Don't get a COVID-19 vaccine if you had a serious allergic reaction, myocarditis, or pericarditis after receiving a *previous* COVID-19 vaccine or any vaccine that contains the same ingredients. It is likely that you will be able to receive a different COVID-19 vaccine if you have had a reaction to one, since the components of the vaccines are not the same. If you've ever had a reaction to any vaccine, be sure to talk to your provider before getting a COVID-19 vaccine.

Any other conditions — even those that are chronic, terminal, or otherwise serious — usually don't prevent you from safely getting the COVID-19 vaccine.

In fact, if you have a medical condition that impairs your immune system, you have an even better reason to get the vaccine because you're more likely to get very sick if you do get COVID-19. For example, contracting COVID-19 during pregnancy increases the risk that you experience adverse outcomes, such as premature birth or stillbirth. Getting vaccinated before or during pregnancy significantly reduces these risks. Talk to your doctor to discuss options.

When to get vaccinated

Get vaccinated as soon as you safely can. I know I don't know everything, but I'm pretty sure I've never seen a 5-month-old baby read — so I can say with confidence that if you're reading this book, you're eligible. Even if you already contracted and recovered from COVID-19, get vaccinated. Vaccination helps prevent COVID from making you super sick in the future, and it makes you less likely to end up in the hospital or to die from COVID-19.

Going for the boosters

If you already got your vaccine, make sure to keep up with new variations and boosters as soon as they come out. Although they're not as common as flu shots yet, COVID-19 vaccines and boosters could become an annual or biannual routine. As researchers and scientists discover more about how to keep us all effectively protected from the virus, our options evolve — so keep your eyes open and stay current! For example, you can check out the CDC and WHO websites for updated information, as well as the website of your local health department.

If you don't stay updated with your booster shots (which boost immune response to existing and new variants) when you need them, you triple your risk of getting infected with COVID-19, according to findings by researchers at Yale School of Public Health and the University of North Carolina at Charlotte published in the January 2023 *Journal of Virology*.

According to the CDC, here's how specific groups can stay updated on their COVID-19 vaccines:

>> **People between 6 years old and 64 years old** should get one bivalent Pfizer-BioNTech or Moderna COVID-19 vaccine.

>> **People who are 65 and older** may get a second dose of the bivalent Pfizer-BioNTech or Moderna COVID-19 vaccine.

>> **Moderately or severely immunocompromised people** may get additional doses of the bivalent Pfizer-BioNTech or Moderna COVID-19 vaccine.

>> **Children who are 6 months old to 5 years old** may need multiple doses of a COVID-19 vaccine to be fully protected, including at least one dose of the bivalent Pfizer-BioNTech or Moderna COVID-19 vaccine, depending on the number of doses they previously received and their age.

Continuing to Mask Up

Regardless of your vaccination or current health status, wearing a mask provides an excellent way to keep yourself and others healthy. Even if you're vaccinated, you can still get (and spread) COVID-19. Wearing a mask adds an extra layer of protection, particularly if you're around others who may have symptoms of COVID-19 — or any other respiratory illness, for that matter.

REMEMBER

Keeping your COVID-19 vaccination current significantly lowers your risk of getting or spreading COVID-19.

Not many silver linings of the pandemic exist, but mainstream social acceptance of masking is one of them — because overall, it helps us all stay healthier by lowering the rate of transmission of all germs that can cause respiratory diseases.

Facts about wearing a mask

Masking reduces the chance of spreading or contracting COVID-19, whether you're wearing cloth masks or medical-grade masks. When you cough or sneeze, you emit large droplets, which the material of almost any type of mask effectively catches, preventing you from transmitting COVID through droplets. Masks even help prevent you from transmitting COVID-19 in aerosol form because aerosols start out as droplets. (See Chapter 5 for more about transmitting the virus through droplets and aerosols.)

When droplets dry out, they leave behind residue, and that residue travels through the air as aerosols. However, as long as the droplets stay trapped in your mask, they remain wet and never dry out enough to become aerosols.

You should wear a mask around others when you

>> Have any respiratory symptoms and haven't been tested for COVID-19 yet.

>> Know that you're positive for COVID-19.

>> Are around others who have tested positive for COVID-19 or display respiratory symptoms.

>> Have an underlying health condition that interferes with the effectiveness of your immune system.

Note: After antibody testing became available (and before vaccines), the medical community discovered that masked hospital healthcare workers were actually less likely to have had COVID-19 than the population at large. This is another testament to the effectiveness of masking.

Keep a collection of masks by your door so that you can grab one on the way out the door, even if you don't think you'll need it. Personally, I've found myself in many situations where I was glad to have a mask to slip on in a crowd.

Choosing a mask

The WHO recommends wearing one of the following types of masks:

>> Disposable medical masks labeled with any of these certifications (which come from various organizations such as American Society for Testing and Materials and the USFDA):

- ASTM F2100
- EN 14683
- YY 0469
- YY/T 0969
- GB 19083
- ASTM F3502

>> Non-medical washable masks that comply with one of these standards:

- ASTM F3502
- CEN/TS17553

You can also wear other masks, as long as they fit you well and have filtration, and you can breathe while wearing them.

Considering mask fit and effectiveness

REMEMBER

Here's a list of different types of masks, in order from most to least effective:

>> **Masks with respirators:** Well-fitting U.S. National Institute for Occupational Safety and Health (NIOSH)–approved masks that include respirators, such as N95s (the U.S. standard for respirators). NIOSH regulates these masks effectively in terms of quality.

>> **Surgical masks:** Well-fitting disposable surgical masks and KN95s (the Chinese standard for respirators). One word of caution here: No one has a reputable certification system for KN95s.

Surgical masks are great for preventing large droplets from spreading, but they don't protect against all germs because they tend to be loose-fitting. Be sure to choose a size that fits your face well and use the wire nose clip if the mask has one.

>> **Tight-weave masks:** Layered, finely woven masks, usually made of cotton, but you can also use silk or flannel.

>> **Loose-knit masks:** These masks are like tight-weave masks but are looser. They aren't as effective as tight-weave masks, but they're better than nothing.

When you decide on a cloth mask

TIP

You can wear a cloth mask over a surgical mask to add extra protection.

Here are some other tips for selecting the right mask:

>> Look for a mask that feels comfy.
>> Choose a style that you like.

>> Make sure that the mask doesn't have any gaps around your nose, mouth, or chin.

>> Choose one that you can wash and dry without damaging it or changing its shape.

You can even make your own mask! Just make sure it has three layers of fabric:

>> **The inner layer:** An absorbent fabric, such as cotton

>> **The middle layer:** Non-woven, non-absorbent material, such as polypropylene

>> **The outer layer:** Non-absorbent material, such as polyester

Caring for your mask

Take your mask off when you get home or when it gets damp. Follow the manufacturer's instructions for handling the mask. And follow these steps for mask care:

1. **Remove your mask by using the ear loop or ties.**

   Don't touch the front cloth part of the mask because that's where all of the germs collect.

2. **If the mask is disposable, throw it out.**

   If it's reusable, remove and dispose of the filter (if it has one).

3. **Throw the used reusable mask right into your clothes washing machine.**

   Or place it in a basin of hot water that contains soap or detergent, if you have to hand-wash the mask.

4. **After cleaning the mask, hang it to air dry.**

5. **Before you wear the mask again, take the extra time to inspect it.**

   Look for any wear and tear, such as holes or thinning material. If you see any damage, if the mask or straps look stretched out, or if you notice stubborn stains or dampness, get rid of the mask.

CASE STUDY: CLOTH MASKS WORKED IN SPRINGFIELD, MISSOURI

In May 2020, two symptomatic hairstylists continued to work while waiting for their COVID-19 tests results. They both wore double-layered cloth masks. They served 139 clients during this time and frequently interacted with coworkers. Throughout the following two-week period, no clients or coworkers tested positive for COVID-19. Considering that they worked indoors in very close contact with both clients and coworkers, this example illustrates how well-layered cloth masks help to prevent the spread of COVID-19.

You can read the report by going to www.cdc.gov, entering "absence of apparent transmission" in the Search text box, and pressing the Search button. The report, titled "Absence of Apparent Transmission of SARS-CoV-2 from Two Stylists After Exposure at a Hair Salon with a Universal Face Covering Policy — Springfield, Missouri, May 2020," should appear in the results. This report appeared in an online article in the CDC's *Morbidity and Mortality Weekly Report (MMWR)* on July 17, 2020.

Evaluating Indoor Ventilation and Outdoor Venues

Because COVID-19 numbers were significantly reduced when the WHO declared the pandemic officially over in May 2023, you don't have to worry about indoor ventilation as much as you did at the height of the pandemic. If you're outside, you definitely don't need to mask because the fresh, moving air disperses aerosols and droplets quickly and effectively.

TIP

If you're hosting an outdoor tented event, use a tent that's as open as possible. The fewer walls the tent has, the better the circulation, which means you greatly reduce the risk of COVID-19 transmission.

And the risks of attending indoor events aren't as potentially devastating as they used to be, thanks to vaccines. However, if your area has an increase in COVID-19 cases, you may find yourself concerned about proper indoor ventilation. That concern is perfectly understandable.

If you have to spend any length of time indoors with others (even briefly) and want to reduce your chances of transmitting or contracting COVID-19, make sure that the room is well-ventilated. Here are some clues that it is:

>> The air doesn't feel stuffy or humid; it feels light and clear.

>> The windows and/or doors are open and letting in air from the outdoors. Open windows across the room from one another is a sign of extra good ventilation because they generate a cross-breeze.

>> The air is moving, either because of a natural breeze from outside or because of fans or other HVAC systems.

>> You see air filtration systems operating around the indoor space.

>> No fans in the room are blowing air so that it moves from one person to another.

TIP

If people in the room are closely spaced, and if anyone is singing or shouting, take extra steps to stay safe, such as socially distancing and wearing a mask, even if you're inside for just a moment. You can still catch COVID-19 during a quick encounter.

Always have a mask on your person! Because masks are so small and lightweight (and available in so many styles, materials, and fits), you can easily stick one or two in your pocket, bag, or car anytime you go out, just in case you need one.

CASE STUDY: CHOIR PRACTICE SUPERSPREADER EVENT IN SKAGIT COUNTY, WASHINGTON

In March 2020, 61 unmasked people attended a two-and-a-half-hour choir practice where one member was symptomatic. Within a week, the local health department identified 53 cases, including 3 people who were hospitalized and 2 who died. During practice, members sat close to one another and shared snacks, in addition to touching the same surfaces, such as chairs. Their singing most likely transmitted COVID-19 via aerosols, which travel farther the more forcefully the lungs expel air (such as when singing). Additionally, some choir members probably emitted more aerosol particles while singing or talking than average because singers are trained in breathing deeply and projecting their voices (and therefore air) stronger than non-singers. This case provides an excellent example of just how quickly people can spread SARS-CoV-2 in certain unique activities and circumstances — especially when no one wears a mask.

You can find the report about this incident at www.cdc.gov. In the Search text box, enter "choir practice," and then click the Search icon. The report titled "High SARS-CoV-2 Attack Rate Following Exposure at a Choir Practice — Skagit County, Washington, March 2020" should appear in the search results. The *Morbidity and Mortality Weekly Report (MMWR)* published the full report on May 15, 2020.

Taking Ongoing Preventative Measures

Here are some things that you can do to help keep the virus from spreading:

>> Stay 6 feet or more away from people other than those in your household when in a crowd indoors.

>> Wear a mask when you are symptomatic or are around others who are.

>> Wash your hands often, using soap and water, for at least 20 seconds each time.

>> Use hand sanitizer if you don't have access to soap and water.

>> Spend as little time as possible in poorly ventilated indoor places with other people (indoor spaces that have open windows, doors, or high-quality ventilation systems pose less risk of transmission).

Practicing good hygiene

Far and away, the most practical hygiene practice for keeping you from getting infections is washing your hands regularly by using soap and water. (If you don't have soap and water available, you can use hand sanitizer.) But how often should you wash your hands? And after or before which activities should you wash them?

A lot of people have a lot of opinions about handwashing, but here are some general guidelines. Whenever possible, wash your hands before touching your face. Also, wash your hands after

>> Cooking food or eating. (Also wash your hands before and during preparing and eating food.)

>> Arriving in a new place.

>> Coughing, sneezing, or blowing your nose.

>> Coming into contact with someone else's respiratory droplets.

>> Using the bathroom.

>> Being around kids or sick people.

>> Playing with a pet.

Not all of the tips in the preceding list deal exclusively with COVID-19 transmission, but the more often you wash your hands in a day, the more you prevent spreading or contracting the SARS-CoV-2 virus (or other germs).

Another good hygienic practice has you step away from others if you need to cough or sneeze — and cover the eruption with the inside of your elbow, even if you're wearing a mask. If others around you are coughing or sneezing, also cover your mouth to prevent someone else's droplets from getting into it.

Eating right and keeping up good general health

"Eat right" might seem like pretty basic advice, but the human body is a complicated combination of systems that all rely on each other to function well. In order for your systems to function well, you have to eat and drink the right foods and beverages. I don't go into a detailed nutrition plan because that discussion would fill a whole other book entirely. If you're interested in finding out more about nutrition, consider picking up a copy of *Nutrition For Dummies*, Seventh Edition by Carol Ann Rinzler (Wiley, 2021).

But it doesn't hurt to throw out a few reminders:

>> **Eat a diet that's well-balanced for your own personal needs.** Make sure that you're taking in plenty of whole grains, proteins, and fruits and vegetables — that's how you get so many of the immune-boosting vitamins and nutrients. Getting vitamins and minerals from a good, balanced diet (rather than from pills) is better because you can typically absorb the nutrients from food sources more reliably than you can from supplements. Also, foods provide other beneficial nutrients, fiber, and antioxidants.

>> **Drink a ton of water.** Water is the key to all life. I know, it can sometimes taste boring or make you have to pee too much, but staying well-hydrated keeps everything running smoothly.

>> **Get good sleep, at least seven to eight hours each night.** This advice is easier said than done most days, probably. But rest and sleep play a vital role in helping you stay healthy. Your body goes through a lot in a day and needs sleep to repair and restore itself.

   When you don't get enough sleep, your body systems become overtaxed and can't function at full force, including your immune system. And when your immune system is weak, that opens the door for sickness, including COVID-19.

>> **Stay active.** Whether you run 5 miles a day or walk your dog around the block, just keep moving. Being active keeps your blood circulation and heart healthy, engages your muscles, and gets everything going.

>> **Get sunshine.** Good ol' Vitamin D, which you can get from sunlight, helps you control inflammation and fight infections. If you live in a place that has little sun (such as Seattle or Alaska during the winter), consider taking a Vitamin D supplement.

USING DELIVERY SERVICES

During the height of the pandemic, the use of delivery services of all kinds skyrocketed. The shutdown of dine-in restaurants notwithstanding, delivery allowed people to stay safe, and the same holds true today.

You can order pretty much anything you want or need. If you don't feel good, stay home. If you don't feel sick but just don't want to face potential exposure to others who are, have what you need delivered.

On top of expanding delivery options for a variety of products and industries, the pandemic gave rise to the idea of contactless drop-off, which offers even more protection for everyone. If you're worried about spreading or contracting illness — COVID-19 or otherwise — choose "contactless delivery" on whatever app you're using to place your order. Delivery services know how to drop off an order without interacting with clients. Just make sure that when you order through your app, you include specific instructions about where to place your items.

Chapter 7

Getting Diagnosed

Y ou know the feeling. You get a tickle in your throat. "Okay, no big deal," you think. Then you start sneezing. Then you're suddenly so tired, you need to get in bed immediately. Things are going downhill fast, and you can't deny it: You're sick. While you make yourself some tea and get under a thousand blankets, you start to wonder whether you have just a cold — or something worse: COVID-19.

Because COVID-19 shares so many symptoms with other respiratory illnesses, you can't figure out whether you have it based just on how you feel. (If you want to go over the symptoms of COVID and how they compare to cold and flu symptoms, see Chapter 5.) In the end, the only way that you can know for sure whether you have COVID-19 is to get tested. Until your test results come back, you can take several steps to put yourself on the path to recovery and prevent potentially spreading COVID to others.

In this chapter, I walk you through everything you can do to find out for sure whether you have COVID-19. And you can also discover the steps to take immediately if you test positive.

Testing for COVID-19 (How to Scratch Your Brain Through Your Nose)

You might suspect that you have COVID-19 because you have symptoms; or maybe you know you were around someone else who tested COVID-positive. Or maybe you recently spent time with a group of people at an indoor location that didn't provide good ventilation (and you didn't wear a mask), so you just want to make sure that you didn't contract the virus. Whatever the case, as soon as you have an inkling that you could possibly have COVID-19, test for it.

When the pandemic first began, getting tested for the virus involved a difficult and time-consuming process. Now, testing for COVID-19 is considerably easier — you can find a wide array of tests available through medical providers, and even over the counter. To get tested, you can make an appointment with your medical provider, walk into a pop-up or urgent care clinic, or even take a test that you can obtain from drugstores, grocery stores, or online at-home.

Exploring diagnostic testing

Diagnostic tests can indicate whether you have a current infection, even if you don't have symptoms. You can find many types of diagnostic tests designed to diagnose different infections. But for COVID-19, providers use two main kinds: polymerase chain reaction (PCR) and antigen tests.

PCR tests

The *polymerase chain reaction* (PCR) test is the most accurate option for testing for the presence of genetic material from the virus that causes COVID-19. PCR is a type of test that falls into a category known as a nucleic acid amplification test (NAAT), which checks for genetic material of a germ. NAATs (both powerful and the industry standard) can detect very small concentrations of genetic material (DNA or RNA), such as the SARS-CoV-2 RNA, that other tests (including antigen tests) might miss.

WARNING

PCR tests are so sensitive, they can detect viral RNA (genetic material) even after you're no longer actively ill or contagious — sometimes as long as three months later. If you get a positive result from a PCR test, but you don't have symptoms and had an infection that was less than 90 days ago, use a rapid antigen test (discussed in the following section) to determine whether you are still contagious. The potential for getting a lingering positive result is why you should not use a PCR test as a "test of cure" if you recently had COVID and have gotten better.

The PCR test comes in both the common nasal-swab style or the saliva-collection style (where you can spit into a tube). A medical provider can perform the PCR test for you, or you can administer it yourself at home (more on that in the section "Administering your own test," later in this chapter). The sample you produce (either through swabbing or spitting) gets sent to a lab for analysis.

Rapid antigen tests

Rapid antigen tests (which test for specific proteins) are great for fast results. If you rely on the results of this type of test, remember that a rapid antigen test is less sensitive than a PCR test (see the preceding section). So if you're not near or at peak infection level (about 3-5 days after your first symptoms) when you receive the test, you could potentially test negative even when you're currently infected and contagious.

TIP

If you use a rapid antigen test and get a negative result, either follow up by taking a PCR test or by doing another antigen test one to two days later.

Although the results you get from a rapid antigen test are not as reliable as the results you get from a standard PCR test, you can still use rapid antigen tests with confidence. You can have a medical professional perform a rapid antigen test on you, or you can use an at-home kit (more on your at-home options in the section "Administering your own test," later in this chapter).

Combination tests

You can even get a single test that checks for flu, Respiratory Syncytial Virus (RSV, a seasonal respiratory virus that usually causes mild, cold-like symptoms but can cause severe disease in babies, in the elderly, and in people with compromised immune systems), and COVID-19 all at the same time. This PCR test uses a nasal swab, like the other PCR tests (see the section "PCR tests," earlier in this chapter) and the rapid antigen tests (discussed in the preceding section).

ANTIBODY TESTS

Although medical providers no longer use antibody tests to diagnose COVID-19, you may still hear about them. During the pandemic, doctors used antibody tests to look for the presence of SARS-CoV-2 antibodies in patients. Your body makes antibodies when you have an infection, and those antibodies are specific for the germ that causes the infection, whether that response comes from an actual COVID-19 infection or from the vaccine. Your body may take a week or two to make enough antibodies for the test to detect, and after you have antibodies, they often persist for life. Antibody tests don't provide effective diagnostic information because they show a positive result, whether from a vaccine and/or previous or current actual infection.

You can go to a medical provider to get the test or do the test at home when you obtain a testing kit online from medical facilities or medical laboratories. The at-home test can give you results in about 30 minutes.

Deciding when to test

You can test for COVID-19 every day if you want, but because the world is no longer in the height of the pandemic (which peaked December 2020–January 2021), that's certainly overkill. The right time to test yourself for COVID-19 differs, depending on the exact circumstances. Here's a quick rundown of the situations in which you should take the test:

>> **If you have symptoms,** test right away (flip to Chapter 5 if you need a look at the symptoms).

>> **If you spend time around someone who has COVID-19 or COVID-like symptoms,** even if you're asymptomatic, take a test three to five full days after you last interacted with them.

>> **If you spend time around someone who tests positive for COVID shortly after your interaction,** test yourself immediately. However, if you get a negative result when you test, test yourself again three to five days after the date of your exposure.

» **If you test positive for COVID,** after five days of isolation (which I talk about in the section "Keeping your germs to yourself: Isolating," later in this chapter), take a test to clear yourself (make sure you're not contagious), assuming that you have mild symptoms which are improving, and you haven't had a fever In the past 24 hours.

» **If you plan to visit someone who's immunocompromised or otherwise at risk,** test before visiting that person.

Administering your own test

If you want to give yourself a test at home, you can use a rapid antigen or PCR test. You can find at-home COVID-19 test kits widely available for purchase over the counter, online, and in most drugstores and pharmacies. And check with your health insurance to see whether you can get some tests for free through them.

TIP

Even if you don't need to take a COVID-19 test right now, stock up on whatever free tests you can get. Also, keep more tests on hand than you think you need. That way, you have them available whenever you (or a loved one, neighbor, or visitor) really needs one. Be sure to check the expiration date on the test before you use It.

Knowing how many test kits to have on hand

Although you might think this number is excessive when you're not sick, consider having enough tests on hand for everyone in your family to take two or three tests. This number of tests gives you enough to get you through a worst-case scenario of everyone needing to test repeatedly.

On top of that, you may want to have extra test kits on hand if you plan a gathering, or if you want to give some kits to friends or family members who suddenly need one themselves but don't have any. Or here's an idea — if you test positive, give a test kit as a gift while you do contact tracing (flip to the section "Mitigating the spread: Contact tracing and informing," later in this chapter). "Sorry, I might have given you COVID. But here's a free test!" Maybe it'll help soften the blow?

Choosing home test kits

When selecting an at-home test, consider whether you need fast results. If you do, take a rapid antigen test (see the section "Exploring diagnostic testing," earlier in the chapter). Also consider the following factors:

REMEMBER

>> **Flexibility:** Because the results of a PCR test can remain positive for many weeks (up to 90 days) after your body has effectively eliminated the virus, a rapid antigen test can determine when you're no longer infectious and don't require isolation. Also, if you have symptoms and a positive antigen test, you have COVID, and a PCR is not needed.

>> **Sensitivity:** If you're currently sick and can wait a few days, go with the PCR. It's more sensitive than a rapid antigen test and less likely to miss diagnosing an infection if you have one.

>> **Sample collection:** Think about which method of test sample collection you can more easily do: swabbing your nasal cavity or spitting saliva into a container. Choose your test accordingly.

Following the instructions for your test kit

Your test kit comes in a box that contains all of the supplies that you need, including instructions. Lay out your materials and read the instructions, then slowly execute the steps while you read through them again. Each test has different instructions, but in general, you either swab or spit:

>> **Most rapid antigen test kits:** Use nasal swabs, which means you swab inside your nose with the kit's swab and place that swab in a tube that contains liquid. You then follow the instructions to determine whether the test is positive.

>> **At-home PCR test kit:** Uses either a nasal swab or your saliva for the test sample. If you have a saliva test kit, simply spit into the included tube and secure the cap. Then follow the instructions for sending it to the lab for processing.

Getting tested in a healthcare setting

You can have a healthcare professional perform your COVID-19 test (free of charge still, in most areas). Some locations are walk-in (such as urgent care facilities and pharmacies), while some require appointments (such as your primary care provider). You can even use a drive-through service at some venues.

To find a facility, do an online search or call your primary care provider, the local health department, or even a local hospital or urgent care. They should all have a list of options for you. They may ask you a few questions to get a sense of your needs, such as

>> Are you experiencing any symptoms?

>> Have you been exposed to COVID-19?

>> Have you recently traveled?

After you find a facility, here's what to expect from the PCR or rapid antigen test that they perform, depending on how they collect a sample:

>> **The swabbing:** Your medical provider inserts a long swab into one nostril to take a sample from the back of your nose. They move the swab around in circles for 15 seconds, and then repeat the process with the other nostril.

- *If the test is a PCR test,* they then put the swab into a secure and labeled container for transport to the lab.

- *If the test is a rapid antigen test,* the next steps vary depending upon the manufacturer. They may put the swab into a small tube of liquid for a minute or more, and then squeeze a few drops of the liquid onto a test stick. Or they may insert a small strip of test paper into the tube of liquid, and after several minutes, see if the strip indicates a positive or negative.

>> **The spitting:** You may have the option to give your provider a saliva sample by spitting into a tube that they provide, which they then secure and label for the lab.

You get your results from PCR tests in one to three days. Even though getting your PCR test results from a medical professional takes a little extra time than getting results from an at-home rapid test, you get more accurate results from the lab. If they give you a rapid antigen test, you get results in about 15 minutes.

WARNING

In the early days of the pandemic, medical professionals used throat swabs to diagnose COVID-19, but the medical community has since figured out that nasal swabs provide more accurate results. I don't recommend using a throat swab because they are not as accurate, so don't submit a sample to testing that you collect this way.

Understanding test results

You complete your test, and now the moment of truth arrives: Are you positive or negative for COVID-19? That question sounds simple enough to answer, but we all know that false negatives and false positives emerge from time to time. So, what's a person to do? Although no testing can guarantee 100 percent foolproof, absolutely correct results, the medical world feels very confident in the effectiveness and accuracy of results of COVID-19 testing.

How you get tested determines how and when you get results:

>> **If a medical professional performs your PCR test for you,** or if you do a home PCR test which is sent to a lab, you most likely get the results in an e-mail or in a text message within one to two days, after the lab processes your sample.

>> **If you take an at-home test,** follow the instructions in the test kit to read your results properly. You can read most kit tests easily, and you probably won't have any questions. But if you're unsure, contact your doctor or other medical provider.

Responding to a Positive Test

You tested positive for COVID-19. Now what? First, remain calm so that you can focus on taking care of yourself and recovering. Next, prevent spreading COVID-19 to other people. Now that COVID has been around since late 2019/early 2020, medical researchers have plenty of data to use to come up with tried-and-true guidance about how to respond to a positive COVID-19 test. Even though the guidance may change a little in response to the natural evolution of the virus, you can follow the advice in the following sections with confidence (unless otherwise instructed by a medical provider).

PCR tests can give positive results for up to three months after a COVID-19 infection, so if you have a positive PCR but recently had COVID-19 and recovered — rest easy. You're not contagious and can go on with your life.

Opting for early treatment

As soon as you get your positive test results, talk to your medical provider about getting treatment for COVID-19. Don't wait for your symptoms to get worse. Getting treatment from a licensed medical provider within five to seven days of diagnosis can significantly reduce your chances of getting very sick, either in the short term or long term.

Anyone 12 years of age or older can take the commonly prescribed medications to treat COVID-19, which you may even get free of charge through funding from the U.S. Department of Health and Human Services. Not everyone who has COVID-19 qualifies for free treatment, but if you are immunocompromised, are a senior, or have pre-existing conditions, you should ask your healthcare providers if you are eligible. Flip to Chapter 8 for more details about the different types of medications available and how to get them.

Keeping your germs to yourself: Isolating

Whether you have symptoms or not, if you test positive for COVID-19, isolate immediately for at least five full days. *Isolating* means you stay in your house, in a room away from other people in your household. Don't go to work or school, don't travel, don't go out and run errands. You don't want to come face to face with anyone at all unless you (and preferably they, too) are wearing a mask.

Facing the aloneness

If you feel lonely when isolating, stay in touch with friends and family however you can. Call and text your loved ones, and video chat so that you can see their faces. If you share a house with others, you can talk through the door or even pass notes back and forth. Try to make a game out of the communication to keep your spirits up. You can also have contact with others if both you and the exposed person wear masks and you maintain a distance of 6 feet from the other person.

If you're alone and need help with getting food or other supplies, dial 311 on your phone to access your city's municipal resources. Although not every single area has 311, the great majority of communities in the U.S. and Canada do. If you're a senior, you can access nonprofits like Meals on Wheels, which provide hot meals to homebound seniors living alone. If you aren't a senior, Project Angel Food can help, or you can do a web search for "delivery services for homebound people" to find other smaller, local nonprofits that provide services to more homebound folks, regardless of age!

Counting the days

To count your five days, make Day 0 the day that you first experienced symptoms or felt sick. Count the next day as Day 1, and so on. If you don't have symptoms and feel fine, Day 0 is the day that you tested positive. You can stop isolating on Day 6, as long as you satisfy both of these requirements:

» Your symptoms are gone, or are mild and improving.

» You haven't had a fever for 24 hours without the aid of medicine.

If Day 5 comes and both of these conditions aren't true, you must continue to isolate until they are. After isolation, you can take an antigen test to make sure you're negative. If your antigen test comes back negative, you can end your isolation and go out and about while masked. See more about masking in the following section.

If you're immunocompromised, you may remain infectious for longer than 5 days or even 10 days. Make sure that you continue to test and follow isolation guidance until you test negative.

Regardless of immune status, if you don't start to feel better after 10 days of isolation, speak to your medical provider. You may be battling Long COVID (flip to Chapter 9 for more on that form of the disease) or other complications.

Masking and keeping your distance

If you can't fully isolate or avoid being around others after you test positive for COVID-19, wear a mask and socially distance yourself as much as possible until Day 10 (assuming that you don't have another positive test), including while inside your own home. For added protection, the others in your home should wear masks, as well.

If you can fully isolate, after you finish with isolation (which you can read about in the section "Keeping your germs to yourself: Isolating," earlier in this chapter), continue to wear a mask around all other people and socially distance until Day 10.

If you don't want to mask, you can take two different antigen tests at least two days apart. If both come back negative without a positive result in between, you can stop masking.

For more specifics on how to do an antigen test, see the section "Testing for COVID-19 (How to Scratch Your Brain)," earlier in this chapter.

Even if you get two negative test results, you may still have to mask through Day 10, depending on your place of employment or local health department guidelines.

For help with choosing a mask, check out to Chapter 6.

Mitigating the spread: Contact tracing and informing

After you test positive, time to do some *contact tracing*, which involves letting the people with whom you've had contact in the recent past know about your status. Follow these steps to do your contact tracing:

1. **Make a list of the people you had close contact with prior to knowing that you had COVID-19.**

    What people you notify depends on whether you have symptoms:

    - *If you have symptoms,* include contacts you made from two days before your symptoms began until now.

    - *If you don't have symptoms,* include the people you interacted with from two days before your positive test until now.

        Close contact means having a person in the same room, less than 6 feet from you, and unmasked — which increases their risk of catching COVID-19 from you. For other factors that increase someone's risk of catching COVID-19 from you when you are infected, see Chapter 11.

2. **Contact each person on the list that you make in Step 1 to let them know when you tested positive for COVID-19.**

    If you don't want to tell them yourself, you can report yourself anonymously through a website set up by the National Coalition of STD Directors (www.tellyourcontacts.org). The website notifies your contacts that they've been exposed to SARS-CoV-2, but it doesn't reveal your identity.

3. **Follow any reporting guidelines set out by your place of employment, school, and local health department.**

REMEMBER

There's no shame in testing positive, so let your contacts know as early as possible, and ask them to spread the word as much as they can to their contacts. If you share this information openly and honestly right away, your contacts can take steps to protect themselves and others.

Quarantining when you've been exposed

Regardless of your vaccination status, if you're on the receiving end of contact tracing — that is, one of your close contacts tests positive — test yourself three to five days after your exposure to this contact. Day 0 is the most recent day when you had close contact with the person who tested positive. Day 1 is the next day, so count from there.

If you suspect you may be infected because you don't feel well or have symptoms (I talk about symptoms of COVID-19 in Chapter 5), you can test right away. However, if you get a negative test before the end of the three-to-five-day window, test again at least one day later within that window. If you test positive, follow the guidance for informing others that I provide in the preceding section.

Here are a few other notes about testing:

>> If you had COVID-19 in the last 30 days, you don't need to test unless you have symptoms.

>> If your last COVID-19 infection was in the last 90 days, use an antigen test versus a PCR test because a PCR might show a false positive because of the bits of the virus still in your respiratory tract from the previous infection.

If you test negative within the three-to-five-day window, monitor yourself for symptoms and mask while indoors for 10 days from date of exposure, especially around any high risk or immunocompromised people. If you start to feel sick or have any symptoms, test immediately.

TIP

If you need help counting the days, you can do an online search for "COVID testing and isolation calculator" to find a tool that you can use to figure out the math. The CDC has a good one here: www.cdc.gov/coronavirus/2019-ncov/your-health/isolation.html.

Chapter **8**

Getting Treated

I f you test positive for COVID-19, you might feel anxious on top of feeling physically bad, but I'm here to help you through it. Most people can manage their COVID-19 at home by resting, drinking plenty of fluids, eating right, and sometimes with the help of over-the-counter medications. But if you're doing all of that and still not feeling better (even if you already had COVID-19 or you're vaccinated — or both), you may need more extensive treatment or help from a medical professional.

In this chapter, I take you through how to know when it's time to get yourself to a doctor, find the right facility for your needs, and get treatment so that you can feel better as soon as possible. I also give you insights on what prescription medications can help you treat COVID-19 and what you can expect if you have the most serious symptoms and must be admitted to the hospital for care.

Seeking Medical Care

Many people experience symptoms when they have COVID-19. If you have the common mild symptoms, such as a fever, body aches, a cough, a headache, or congestion, you can probably get through the sickness just fine at home. But if you have any of the more serious symptoms — or any symptoms worsen to the point of becoming severe — get professional medical care. For example, seek help if

>> You struggle to catch your breath or are breathing faster than usual.

>> You feel pain or pressure in your chest.

>> You feel significantly confused, disoriented, or struggle to stay awake.

>> You have bluish lips or face.

>> You struggle to eat or drink.

>> You feel severely fatigued, and the fatigue is getting worse, not better.

>> Your pre-existing chronic medical conditions — such as diabetes or heart disease — worsen.

REMEMBER

Symptoms should get better, not worse. Symptoms occur because your body is fighting infection. While your immune system battles the infection, it should begin to win, and the symptoms should lessen; symptoms should eventually disappear after your immune system wins the battle.

Acting quickly

When you have severe symptoms, or your symptoms worsen, don't wait to seek medical care. Trust your gut — you know when you don't feel right and when something is really wrong with your body. Even if you don't know whether your symptoms are really serious enough to require medical attention, have a doctor check you out. The sooner you get medical intervention, the faster you can stabilize, manage your infection, and prevent potential complications from popping up.

When you receive early intervention for COVID-19, your doctor may provide any combination of supportive care, antiviral medications, and other therapies. We doctors base the treatment you receive on your current individual medical status and the guidelines from your local health department, the Centers for Disease Control and Prevention (CDC; www.cdc.gov), the Infectious Diseases Society of America (IDSA; www.idsociety.org), and other professional organizations.

Knowing where to go for help

When you're feeling bad enough that you need medical attention, you may wonder whether you should make an appointment with your regular doctor or make tracks to the closest urgent care or emergency room. The answer depends primarily on your symptoms:

>> **If you have mild symptoms,** such as low-grade fever, cough, sore throat, or mild body aches, call your regular doctor to set up either an in-person or remote telehealth appointment. After the doctor sees or confers with you, they can tell you whether you need additional care or can get by with at-home care.

>> **If you have moderate to severe symptoms,** such as high fever, difficulty breathing, chest pain, persistent cough, or significant fatigue, go directly to an urgent care or emergency room to get immediate care.

Stay updated about the current COVID-19 practices in your area by checking the websites of local and national public health agencies. Even though guidelines and protocols for seeking COVID-19 medical care have stayed consistent between the time the pandemic officially ended and when I wrote this book, they can change at any time.

TIP

If you can't think clearly enough because you don't feel good, have a loved one help you make the decision about where to get care — and then ask them to drive you there.

Taking Prescribed Medications That Work

In the U.S., you can find proven and safe COVID-19 medications widely available, and most healthy people 12 years and older can take them safely, as long as a medical professional prescribes them. But here's the catch: COVID-19 medications work best when you take them within the first five to seven days after the first onset of your symptoms.

WARNING

Don't use medications outside of a prescription written for you. Using unauthorized medication to treat COVID-19 can cause you problems if you use them in an off-label or unapproved way. During the height of the pandemic, many people experimented with different drugs (such as ivermectin) out of sheer desperation, which was dangerous because it can cause nausea, vomiting, low blood pressure, seizures, and even death.

When you take the right medications as prescribed, they can help you in a number of ways. For example, they can

>> Stop you from getting seriously ill, needing to be hospitalized, or dying from COVID-19.

>> Potentially help you test negative for the virus sooner than if you didn't take the medications.

>> Make you less likely to transmit the virus to others.

You can have serious reactions to any medication or treatment (just like with food or bee stings), and allergic reactions, including anaphylaxis, which can be life-threatening. Alert a medical professional right away if, during your treatment with any medication, you

>> Feel a chill or start shaking.

>> Feel dizzy.

>> Have a headache.

>> Start sweating profusely.

>> Have trouble breathing or swallowing.

>> Start itching or see a rash on your skin.

>> Feel lightheaded or faint.

>> Feel your heart beating fast, unusually strongly, or unevenly.

>> Notice your hands, face, or mouth swelling.

Antivirals

Your healthcare provider may prescribe *antiviral medications* (also called *antivirals*), which help your body decrease the amount of the virus in your blood (otherwise known as *viral load*), as well as help reduce your symptoms.

Regardless of your vaccination status or previous COVID-19 infections, some of the most common complications from COVID-19 that antiviral medications help you avoid are

>> Abnormal heart rhythms

>> Blood clots in lungs

>> Thrombosis

>> Fatigue and malaise

>> Liver disease

>> Acute kidney injury

>> Muscle pain

>> Impaired thinking or reasoning

At the time of this writing, three main COVID-19 antivirals are available to consumers. See the following mini table for their generic, brand, and manufacturer names.

Brand Name	Generic Name	Manufacturer
Veklury	Remdesivir	Gilead Sciences
Paxlovid	Nirmatrelvir/ritonavir	Pfizer
Lagevrio	Molnupiravir	Merck

Veklury (remdesivir)

Scientists originally developed Veklury (remdesivir) to treat Ebola. But they discovered that it was effective in treating some coronaviruses, so the U.S. Food and Drug Administration (FDA) initially authorized it to treat the most severe COVID-19 cases during the pandemic. Medical providers still use it today as a highly effective treatment.

Your doctor may prescribe Veklury for you if you have mild to moderate symptoms of COVID-19 in order to prevent you from becoming sicker and keep you out of the hospital. The specific dosage and treatment duration depends on the severity of your case, any medications that you're taking, and your overall health.

You receive the treatment *intravenously* (as a liquid administered through a catheter placed into one of your veins) while in a medical facility. Here are potential scenarios for treatment with Veklury:

>> **If you are an outpatient,** a healthcare provider inserts a needle into one of your veins and slowly gives you a liquid

form of the medicine over the course of anywhere from 30 minutes to 2 hours. If your infusion goes off without a problem, you can then go home and rest. Your provider will advise you on what time to return the following day.

Usually, you receive one dose a day for three days, coming back to the same medical facility each time.

>> **If you're already hospitalized,** you may receive up to 5 to 10 intravenous doses (administered over time between 30 minutes and 2 hours per dose), at one dose per day.

When you get Veklury treatments, your medical provider monitors you closely to make sure that you respond well and don't have a serious reaction. And if you do have a reaction, they're right there to take care of you.

Always complete your treatment in accordance with your doctor's plan. Don't end after the first dose because the treatment won't work. And definitely don't try Veklury or any other medication unless you're under the care of a physician.

REMEMBER

Give your physician a complete medical history before you begin treatment because Veklury can adversely affect you if you have certain pre-existing conditions, especially kidney disease or liver disease. Also, let them know if you currently take or have recently taken chloroquine or hydroxychloroquine (more on those ineffective treatments in the section "Hydroxychloroquine," later in this chapter).

TIP

After you return home, you should continue to monitor yourself (or ask a loved one to monitor you) for strange or severe side effects. Keep in mind, Veklury can cause common side effects, such as pain or swelling at the IV site, headache, or feeling tired. Talk to your provider about all side effects before you leave the treatment facility so that you know what to expect and how to identify side effects that require medical attention, such as shortness of breath, increased heart rate, sweating, or fever.

Paxlovid (nirmatrelvir/ritonavir)

The history of Paxlovid (nirmatrelvir/ritonavir) begins in 2003 with another antiviral known as PF-00835231. The pharmaceutical company Pfizer developed this antiviral to treat SARS intravenously. Pfizer didn't get to use this medication immediately after they developed it because, by the time the drug was ready for trials, the SARS outbreak was over.

Cut to: March 2020. When the COVID-19 pandemic began, Pfizer's scientists looked back at the drug and made changes so that they could offer a COVID-19–fighting antiviral in pill form. And that's how Paxlovid was born.

Your medical provider may prescribe Paxlovid for you if you have a higher risk than the average person of becoming extremely sick, being hospitalized, or dying from COVID-19. Factors that throw you into this high-risk category (where you're more likely to get a prescription for Paxlovid) include

>> **Your age:** 50 years or older

>> **Vaccination status:** Unvaccinated

>> **Certain medical conditions:** Obesity, chronic lung disease, heart disease, or a weakened immune system, for example

If you're prescribed Paxlovid, you take three pills twice daily for five days. In order for Paxlovid to work at suppressing the SARS-CoV-2 virus, your doctor should have you start Paxlovid as soon as possible after you test positive for COVID-19 and within five days of symptom onset.

REMEMBER

Just like with Veklury (see the preceding section), you need to give your doctor a full medical history (especially if you have liver or kidney disease), including a list of all the medications that you currently take. *Note:* Paxlovid can interact with multiple other meds and possibly cause toxicity — especially with some blood thinning medications, statin drugs (which treat high cholesterol), HIV medications, erectile dysfunction drugs, and hydrocodone.

Here are the common side effects of Paxlovid:

>> **Metallic taste in your mouth:** The main side effect of Paxlovid that you might experience. Although you may have this metallic taste for the full five days of treatment, it should go away after you stop taking the medication.

>> **Gastrointestinal problems:** You may also experience gastrointestinal distress and diarrhea. As long as you don't have severe symptoms, you don't need additional medical attention to treat this side effect.

Lagevrio (molnupiravir)

Researchers at Emory University originally developed Lagevrio (molnupiravir) in 2014 to treat the Venezuelan equine encephalitis virus. After working with the antiviral over the next several years, researchers found that this medication could treat other viruses, including coronaviruses.

In March 2020, when the pandemic started, scientists tested it on SARS-CoV-2 and found that it worked to disrupt virus reproduction by introducing multiple mutations into the virus's *genome* (its complete set of DNA).

Lagevrio became available on an emergency basis as the first oral COVID-19 treatment, and the medical community still uses it effectively today. Although Lagevrio is less effective than Veklury or Paxlovid (discussed in the preceding sections), it's far more effective than taking no medication at all. And your doctor may prescribe it to you when (for some other health reason) you can't take Veklury or Paxlovid.

If you start Lagevrio treatment within five days of your positive COVID-19 test, this medicine can help you recover faster than you would without it — up to four days sooner, in some cases. It can also help keep post-COVID complications and Long COVID at bay. You take Lagevrio orally twice daily for five days to try to keep your mild-to-moderate COVID-19 symptoms from progressing.

You may experience any number of common side effects from the medication, including

>> Diarrhea

>> Nausea

>> Dizziness

WARNING

If you fall into one of the following groups, you have additional drawbacks and concerns of Lagevrio use:

>> **If you can potentially become pregnant,** abstain from sex or use reliable contraception for the duration of treatment and for four days after completing your treatment. If you do become pregnant, Lagevrio can potentially harm your unborn baby, as researchers have not yet studied the effects on unborn babies.

>> **If you can potentially impregnate someone,** abstain from sex with people who can potentially become pregnant or use a reliable method of contraception for the duration of treatment and for at least three months after your last dose — because some medications can remain in semen for that long.

>> **If you're pregnant or lactating,** don't take Lagevrio because scientists have not yet studied the effects of the drug on babies and pregnant women.

>> **If you're younger than 18 years,** don't take Lagevrio because scientists have not yet studied the effects of the drug on those under 18.

REMEMBER

And now for some good news: The FDA has yet to identify any drug-drug interactions with Lagevrio — but still tell your doctor every medication that you're currently taking as part of your medical history before you get your prescription.

Steroids

If you have severe or critical COVID-19, your doctor may prescribe corticosteroids such as dexamethasone to supplement your other treatments. This treatment reduces the likelihood that you'll become unable to breathe well enough on your own, and need to be put on a ventilator to breathe or that you'll die from COVID-19 (among other reasons).

Symptoms of severe COVID-19 include

>> Signs of pneumonia

>> Severe respiratory distress

>> Low blood oxygen level

>> Septic shock

>> Needing life-sustaining treatment to remain stable

REMEMBER

Taking steroids when you have only a mild case can put you at risk for major complications, so if your doctor doesn't give you steroids, don't worry that you're missing a chance to add power to your treatment. In the early stages of COVID-19 or in mild cases, it is important to allow the immune system to fight the virus. Steroids can impair this immune response. If you develop a severe disease, your immune system goes into *overdrive* and can cause more harm than good. Steroids can help you — in these overdrive situations — to avoid complications such as being put on a ventilator or death.

If your doctor administers corticosteroids to you, you may get them through pills or injections over a course of seven to ten days. Medical staff will monitor you closely to make sure that your blood *glucose* (sugar) levels don't increase too much. An increase in blood glucose typically happens when a person takes steroids, but only to a certain level, and it should cease after you finish treatment.

WARNING

You're extra susceptible to complications from steroids if you

>> Have diabetes, cancer, open wounds (following traumatic injuries), severe burns, or malnourishment

>> Take immunosuppressants or immunomodulators to treat cancer or autoimmune diseases

>> Have severe immunodeficiencies

>> Use IV drugs

Avoiding Treatments That Don't Work

Although you may feel tempted to try unapproved drugs and treatments when you're desperate to feel better, don't do it. You put yourself at greater risk by experimenting without the supervision of a physician.

WARNING

Thanks to sanctioned research, the medical community knows a lot about several common treatments that became very popular among the public during the pandemic, and can say with full confidence, DON'T TRY THESE AT HOME!

Hydroxychloroquine

Hydroxychloroquine first appeared in the 1940s as a malaria treatment. Now, doctors also use it to treat autoimmune disorders, such as rheumatoid arthritis and lupus.

During the pandemic, the FDA approved it for emergency use to treat COVID-19. But the medical community found that hydroxychloroquine didn't stop people from getting infected, being hospitalized, needing ventilators, or dying from COVID-19. So, we doctors no longer recommend this medication as a treatment or preventative for COVID-19.

Azithromycin

Azithromycin is an *antibiotic*, which means it fights bacteria. Because COVID-19 is caused by a virus (SARS-CoV-2), azithromycin doesn't actually help or treat your symptoms in any way. It may address other types of infections that you just happen to have at the same time that you're suffering from COVID-19, but it doesn't treat or resolve COVID-19.

Ivermectin

Ivermectin is an *antiparasitic*, which means it kills off parasites in your system. Because SARS-CoV-2 isn't a parasite (it's a virus), ivermectin can't help treat it. Studies of the effect of ivermectin on COVID-19 have revealed that it doesn't shorten the illness, nor keep you out of the hospital.

CONVALESCENT PLASMA

Convalescent plasma is sort of 50/50: Some studies show that it is effective in treating COVID-19, and others indicate that it is not. *Blood plasma* is the liquid part of your blood that doesn't contain blood cells but does contain antibodies. Antibodies form in your immune system when you're infected with a germ and then recover from that infection. Plasma obtained during convalescence is likely to carry antibodies against the virus. Doctors can use that plasma to help treat others who are sick.

In 2020, the FDA granted emergency authorization for doctors to use plasma antibodies as a way to treat COVID-19. However, it got mixed results in clinical trials, and researchers saw that too many variables impact convalescent plasma's effectiveness, making it an inconsistent treatment option. So I don't recommend pursuing this treatment unless you're immunocompromised and your system can't produce its own antibodies.

Opting for OTC Medication Support

If you have mild COVID-19 symptoms, you can recover at home. If you need to, grab some over-the-counter (OTC) drugs to help. They won't actually fight the virus, but they can provide you with some relief from symptoms, which can make you feel better.

TIP

Here's how you can fight some common COVID-19 symptoms by using OTC meds:

>> **Fever or chills:** Take a something in the analgesic class of drugs, like acetaminophen (Tylenol) or something in the non-steroidal anti-inflammatory drug (NSAID) class, like ibuprofen (Motrin/Advil) or naproxen (Advil/Aleve). These medications not only reduce fever, but also reduce that achy feeling that many people get when they have COVID-19. Fever actually helps your body to fight off infection more effectively, so don't treat your fever unless it's causing you serious discomfort.

>> **Cough:** Take a cough suppressant such as Robitussin (dextromethorphan) or an OTC medication that contains guaifenesin, such as Mucinex. *Guaifenesin* is an expectorant; it thins the mucus in your air passages, which helps loosen the mucus in your chest.

Coughing is also one of the ways that the body fights off an infection, just like a fever. Go easy on the cough suppressants and use them only if you have an excessively painful or prolonged cough or one that prevents you from getting a good night's sleep.

>> **Headache:** If the acetaminophen or ibuprofen doesn't do the trick, try aspirin, which may treat headaches better than those medications for some people. You can also take ibuprofen (or aspirin) with acetaminophen (but not with aspirin) if either one doesn't work alone. If you need even more help, you can try a product that has caffeine in it, such as Excedrin.

>> **Sore throat:** Lozenges can help you soothe an irritated or scratchy throat. If your throat is extra painful, choose lozenges that contain *benzocaine,* a local anesthetic that has a numbing effect. And if you have a cough on top of a sore throat, choose lozenges that include a cough suppressant, such as dextromethorphan.

Accepting Hospitalization
When You Need It

You may need to be hospitalized if you have severe symptoms of or complications from COVID-19 that you can't overcome at home by resting and taking medication. These serious issues can include

» **Trouble breathing,** especially while you're simply at rest or doing light activity.

» **Blood oxygen levels below 94 percent,** or lower if you have a pre-existing respiratory condition. Your doctor or an urgent care facility can advise you about an acceptable blood oxygen level.

» **Worsening of pre-existing conditions,** for example, chronic diseases such as heart disease, lung disease, diabetes, and compromised immune systems.

» **Dehydration** because the disease's symptoms or decreased thirst create a situation in which you can't drink enough to stay hydrated.

» **Mental health effects,** such as feeling confused, too tired to stay awake, or otherwise altered mentally.

» **High and persistent fever** (101 degrees Fahrenheit or higher) that does not respond to medication or that lasts for three or more days.

» **Severe and persistent cough** that keeps you awake at night and prevents you from relaxing.

» **Chest pain or pressure** that can signify a heart or lung problem.

» **Bluish lips or face,** which mean that you don't have enough oxygen in your blood, or your blood isn't circulating well.

REMEMBER

Even if you don't have the symptoms in the preceding list but do have a symptom that leaves you feeling really unwell (and nothing you try makes you feel any better), call your doctor to find out whether you need to see a healthcare professional. It's better to be safe than sorry when it comes to COVID-19.

Receiving supportive care

COVID-19 doesn't have a cure, so when you're hospitalized for COVID-19, you get supportive care to help you manage your symptoms, relieve suffering, and stabilize your overall condition. Of course, as noted in the section "Antivirals" earlier in the chapter, antiviral medications may also be an important part of your care.

Although everyone's experience varies slightly depending on location and condition, you follow these general steps if you're hospitalized for COVID-19:

1. **Prepare for an examination by a medical professional.**

   When you arrive at the ER or urgent care facility, medical staff assess you to determine how sick you are and what type of care you need. They take your vital signs (temperature, heart rate, and blood pressure), check your blood oxygen levels, and give you a physical exam. And they might take X-rays of your lungs and run blood tests.

2. **Embrace the necessary isolation.**

   Staff may place you in a private room or designated area for COVID-19 patients to help prevent spreading the virus.

3. **Submit to supportive care.**

   Staff puts you on IV fluids to keep you hydrated, medicates you to manage your fever and cough, and puts you on supplemental oxygen if you have low blood oxygen levels. (See the following section for discussion of oxygenation in the hospital.) They adjust your care while your condition changes.

4. **Transfer to ICU, if needed.**

   If you're not getting better, you get worse, or you arrive at the facility in an extremely critical condition, the staff may transfer you to the Intensive Care Unit (ICU). You may be put on a ventilator or receive *extracorporeal membrane oxygenation* (ECMO), which is a life support machine that oxygenates your blood if your lungs aren't working properly.

5. **Follow your discharge orders.**

   After your condition stabilizes and your doctor feels that you're doing well enough to safely function at home on your own without supplemental medical treatment, the hospital releases you with instructions for managing your symptoms from home and isolating there if you need to.

Undergoing oxygenation

If your blood oxygen levels are below 94 percent saturation, but your lungs are still functioning normally, you may need supplemental oxygen and breathing help in some form. Getting this extra oxygen temporarily can help you stabilize and re-oxygenate your blood to get it back to normal, healthy blood oxygen levels. For example, the oxygen treatment may go something like this, from least to most intensive:

» **Nasal tube:** You may receive the oxygen through a tube that goes under your nose, loops over your ears, and pushes oxygen into your nostrils. Your medical provider can adjust the flow, as needed.

» **Face mask:** If supplemental oxygen through a tube doesn't effectively raise your blood oxygen levels, the medical staff may give you oxygen through a face mask that covers your mouth and nose.

» **High flow:** If the face mask doesn't do the trick, oxygen may be given using *high flow* (a setup that includes a large nasal cannula), which delivers much higher concentrations of oxygen that have been warmed and humidified.

» **Ventilator:** If your lungs still can't seem to provide your blood with enough oxygen, doctors may put you on a *ventilator,* a device that breathes for you and takes over the work of your lungs so that they can rest and recover.

Riding out the Course of the Virus and Recovering

Regardless of the symptoms that you experience and treat while you're suffering from COVID-19, be kind to yourself and don't rush into activities or overdo it. You may feel like you're missing out on work or play — or maybe you're even getting pressure from others to hurry up and feel better. If you need guidance for advocating for yourself and your rights in the workplace, turn to Chapters 9 and 11. Tune out any inner (or outer) voices and just let yourself fully rest.

Take as many naps as you need, for as many days as you need. If you try to shortcut the recovery process, you just wind up being sick for longer (or becoming sick again). On average, if you're healthy and vaccinated, you should feel better in about one or two weeks.

Keeping yourself healthy and entertained

At this point in the evolution of COVID-19, most cases are mild to moderate, so you most likely can recover from your infection at home pretty quickly. See Chapter 7 for what to do after you test positive to make sure that you keep yourself and others safe. To keep yourself comfortable while you wait for your immune system to reduce or eliminate the SARS-CoV-2 virus from your system, here are some tips:

>> Keep plenty of your favorite electrolyte solutions (such as Gatorade or coconut water, and Pedialyte for children) stocked up, and keep hydrating!

>> Stay on a regular schedule when you take any over-the-counter (OTC) meds. Don't let too much time pass between doses, otherwise you risk letting your symptoms creep up again, making you feel even lousier.

>> If you're feeling well enough to be bored, find quiet activities or hobbies that can entertain you while you're sick, such as listening to audiobooks or reading, binge watching that show you've been wanting to catch up on, or talking on the phone.

Ask friends or family members to make no-contact deliveries of new puzzle books, magazines, or newspapers to keep your supply of distractions fresh.

>> Splurge on delivery! If you lose your sense of taste or smell because of COVID-19 (which I talk about in Chapter 9), you may not feel much like eating, but try to force yourself to keep your nutrition up. Order from your favorite places to try to coax your appetite out.

Dealing with factors that complicate recovery

Sometimes, you may not recover as well as others if you have certain conditions or other factors influencing your immune system and overall health. Even if you feel okay and like you can manage recovery by yourself at home, monitor yourself for any sudden or severe changes. Get to a doctor right away if you notice anything amiss (see the section "Seeking Medical Care," earlier in this chapter, for a list of severe symptoms to watch out for).

Be prepared to take action quickly if you

>> Have any pre-existing chronic or autoimmune conditions or are immunocompromised

>> Are 65 years or older

>> Are unvaccinated

>> Are obese, diabetic, or have kidney, lung, or liver disease

Chapter 9

Managing Long COVID

By some estimates, Long COVID — also known by other names (some of which are scary), including *long-haul COVID*, *post-acute COVID-19*, *post-acute sequelae of SARS-CoV-2 infection/PASC*, or *chronic COVID* — affects up to 45 percent of all people worldwide who have recovered from COVID-19, but continue to have at least one unresolved symptom. This statistic was reported in the article "The prevalence and long-term health effects of Long Covid among hospitalised and non-hospitalised populations: a systematic review and meta-analysis" by Lauren L. O'Mahoney et al, in the December 1, 2022 issue of *The Lancet*.

Long COVID remains a bit of a mystery, even to medical providers and researchers. The science and medical communities debate about which symptoms comprise Long COVID, and how long those symptoms last. For the purposes of this book, *Long COVID* refers to any COVID-19 symptoms — mild, severe, or anything in between —that recovery from your initial COVID-19 infection hasn't resolved. (See Chapter 5 for more information about being contagious.)

The medical community can't easily compare Long COVID to other post-viral illnesses because no other virus has been as widespread and impactful as COVID-19. In this chapter, I share what the medical community knows about Long COVID as of the writing of this book. But fortunately, researchers have probably already discovered more details by the time you read this book.

Knowing Whether You're Likely to Develop Long COVID

For the good news first, scientists are noticing that new cases of Long COVID seem milder than those that occurred during the pandemic. They don't fully understand why later cases of Long COVID are relatively mild, but two prevailing theories are

» More people are fully vaccinated against the virus, and the vaccine has been shown to reduce the risk of getting Long COVID.

» The recent COVID-19 variants aren't as strong as the original strain, so the infection doesn't cause as many severe symptoms.

Scientists still have a lot to learn about Long COVID; however, some findings emerge consistently in their studies and indicate that certain factors may make you more likely to develop Long COVID, including

» **Your immune system overreacts to a COVID-19 infection.** To fight off infection, your body produces immune cells that launch an attack against the virus. After your immune system destroys the virus, it's supposed to stop — but sometimes it doesn't. It may keep going, even though you don't need it anymore. This overreaction can cause prolonged inflammation, which can lead to tissue damage that can cause Long COVID symptoms to set in, such as difficulty breathing and cognitive decline.

» **Your body holds virus reservoirs.** Another theory suggests that the COVID-19 virus may collect and hide out in different tissues, organs, or cells. These reservoirs can become active and trigger you to have ongoing symptoms and flare-ups.

» **Before you got COVID-19, you had pre-existing health conditions,** such as heart disease, diabetes, or obesity.

» **You're a biological female.** Some studies have suggested that this population is at greater risk than biological males, and they're up to twice as likely to of develop ongoing symptoms — such as fatigue, shortness of breath, brain fog, muscle pain, anxiety, or depression — after their initial COVID-19 infection. Also, women are more prone to autoimmune disease, in general, which COVID-19 can exacerbate. If you're a woman aged 40 to 60 years old, you can be at even more risk than people who are outside of that age group and gender.

>> **You had more than five symptoms during the first week of your COVID-19 infection.** According to data collected from the *Zoe Health Study app* (which people can download from https://health-study.joinzoe.com/app and use to track and report their COVID-19 symptoms), people who experienced more symptoms during their COVID-19 infection are 3.5 times more likely to develop Long COVID than are people who had fewer COVID symptoms during infection.

>> **You had a high viral load during your COVID-19 infection.** According to research published in the peer-reviewed journal *Cell*, people who had higher amounts of the virus in their bodies during the early stages of infection were more likely to develop persistent symptoms, maybe because they had more of the virus to start with and/or their bodies couldn't control the infection after it got started.

>> **You have too many *autoantibodies*.** At the time of your COVID-19 infection, you may have an autoimmune disease that leads to having too many antibodies that attack your body's healthy tissue, instead of going after intruders such as viruses. The more these autoantibodies multiply and activate, the fewer SARS CoV-2 antibodies your body makes. Without those early antibodies to battle COVID-19, the disease may set in for the long haul.

>> **Your gut microbiome was (or still is) unbalanced.** The gut *microbiome* is the collection of microorganisms, such as bacteria and fungi, that live in your GI tract. These microorganisms in your intestines may influence how well your body responds to viruses and bacteria. People who have variations, mutations, or a simple imbalance in their gut may be more at risk for many diseases and be more likely to get Long COVID. Our knowledge of the intestinal microbiome is at a very early stage, as is our understanding of its role in

disease. But you can expect to hear much more about the microbiome in the near future.

>> **You're unvaccinated against COVID-19.** Multiple studies show evidence that being vaccinated reduces or totally eliminates the length of time you have Long COVID. Some studies show that, even if you don't get vaccinated until after your infection, the vaccine may still reduce your chances of getting Long COVID.

>> **You've had COVID-19 multiple times.** Reinfections make you more susceptible to Long COVID's unresolved symptoms.

REMEMBER

Anyone can get Long COVID. Some people get Long COVID without having pre-existing illness or underlying conditions, and the medical community doesn't know enough yet to understand why. Scientists are still researching to find out more about what precipitates Long COVID.

Uncovering health inequities

Some population groupings or communities around the world — particularly in the U.S. — face health disparities, inadequate healthcare infrastructure, and other inequities because of systemic racism, classism, homophobia, or even incarceration status. When you face these types of obstacles, you're more at risk of contracting Long COVID.

COVID infection rates — as well as complications and Long COVID — are higher in *marginalized populations* (the groups that experience discrimination and exclusion in society). The CDC estimates that some *BIPOC* (Black, indigenous, and people of color) populations experience hospitalization after COVID-19 infection at a rate more than threefold higher than non-marginalized communities. These marginalized communities are also more likely to be unvaccinated and to have inadequately treated medical conditions such as diabetes and heart disease, making them more susceptible to COVID-19 and to Long COVID.

Adversities faced by marginalized communities

Because of lifelong inadequate healthcare, pre-existing conditions tend to disproportionally affect marginalized communities, including

- » Autoimmune disease
- » Cardiovascular disease
- » Chronic respiratory disease
- » Diabetes
- » Hypertension
- » Liver disease
- » Obesity

And these factors can adversely affect the access to and affordability of adequate nutrition and healthcare. People in marginalized populations

- » **Are more likely to be essential workers** and, therefore, less likely to work remotely. As a result, they're more likely to come into contact with contagions.

- » **Often live in higher-density environments** and can't always isolate at home when they have symptoms because they're more likely to live in multigenerational households with more people.

- » **Under-test and under-vaccinate** because of distrust of the medical field as a result of decades of racist actions and policies. (See the sidebar "The Tuskegee syphilis study," in this chapter, to find out about one of the most infamous examples.)

- » **Face discrimination, cultural insensitivity, and unconscious bias** from providers. They sometimes can't access medical services in their native language. And they often don't have access to quality health insurance.

- » **Don't always have access to quality (or any) medical providers** near where they live. They're less likely to have reliable transportation to get to medical care facilities and often have to rely on public transportation, limiting their medical-care options.

- » **May have access to inadequately funded facilities** that don't have updated equipment, or enough staff or beds available.

- » **Often face food insecurity, food deserts, and other factors** that contribute to undernourishment, diabetes, and hypertension.

THE TUSKEGEE SYPHILIS STUDY

From 1932 to 1972, in Tuskegee, Alabama, the U.S. Public Health Service (USPHS) ran an unethical and highly damaging experiment on Black people, rooted in racism, to determine how syphilis behaves naturally.

They didn't fully inform nor obtain consent from study participants, who believed that they were receiving treatment for their already-existing syphilis. Instead, researchers allowed the disease to run its course unchecked and untreated. Even after they developed a treatment (penicillin), the government didn't offer it to study participants.

The white researchers of the USPHS justified this study by saying Black people would never agree to get treatment for syphilis. They sold their racist experiment to the public as an observation of the natural progression of syphilis within a community that refused to seek treatment. And those researchers got away with their lie and continued their study for 40 years. Some reports note Black men lost an average of 1.4 years off of their life expectancy because of this study, to say nothing of the devastating mental and emotional trauma that this community continues to suffer because of it.

The program was finally ended in 1972 after a news story about the study spurred a review. In the summer of 1973, the participants brought a class action lawsuit against the U.S. government, which they won; but nothing can ever undo the damage the USPHS did. And this study presents just one example that illustrates why marginalized communities have severe and justified mistrust of medical care.

REMEMBER

All of these obstacles make it hard for people to access medical services, even when they need them — including when they're sick with COVID-19, which increases their chances of experiencing Long COVID. These obstacles also make it much less likely that marginalized communities get the COVID-19 vaccine, which may be the single most effective preventive measure against Long COVID.

Initiating positive reform in marginalized communities

If you are BIPOC (Black, Indigenous, or person of color) or a member of other marginalized communities, you may be able to access financial assistance and other resources to help you recover from and live with Long COVID. The Center for Urban and Racial Equity, for example, has a mutual aid network (at https://urbanand racialequity.org/hub_category/mutualaid/) that includes many options for COVID help.

Although many initiatives from the U.S. federal government attempt to improve access to care and expand insurance coverage for the most at-risk communities, people who can obtain this insurance often face sky-high insurance copayments and deductibles, prescription costs, and monthly premiums. Many people find it almost impossible to receive the care that they need, when they need it.

Avoiding Long COVID

Because we in the medical community are still very much learning about Long COVID, no one has any absolute surefire proven methods to prevent Long COVID. But we have seen some practices that may possibly help, such as

THE RISK OF LONG COVID FOR THOSE WHO ARE INCARCERATED

A paper published in the National Library of Medicine in August 2021 states, "[T]he case rate for COVID-19 for incarcerated individuals is 5.5 times higher than the nonincarcerated population and death rate is 3 times higher than the nonincarcerated population."

Someone who's incarcerated has a high likelihood of experiencing Long COVID because of the environment in which they live: so many people all packed together in a small, indoor location for most of every day, which means viruses can very easily and quickly spread. Also, many incarcerated people have pre-existing health conditions, and people with these conditions living in that environment have an extremely high risk of infection because ventilation is poor (meaning germs in the air don't move on or filter as easily as they do in open air), the population is dense (making transmitting germs between people much easier), and their stress level is high (which lowers their immune system's ability to fight viruses and bacteria).

ON THE HORIZON: MEDICATIONS TO PREVENT LONG COVID?

Aside from maintaining your personal health and wellness, you may soon be able to turn to medication to help keep you from developing Long COVID. Multiple research teams are studying how several different drugs can potentially help prevent Long COVID. (As of the publishing of this book, the world still doesn't have an approved prevention medication.)

Part of the challenge of finding effective drug-based prevention (and treatment) options for Long COVID is that the symptoms are so varied from person to person. Some scientists are grouping similar symptoms together and treating different groups in different ways to see whether that approach works. It's likely that treatment for Long COVID won't be a one-size-fits-all approach. We doctors will continue to base treatment on the specific symptoms (what the patient tells them) and signs (findings on examination). The medical community has the drive and desire to find a solution; it's only a matter of time before they find it.

» Getting a COVID-19 infection treated early

» Maintaining good nutrition

» Doing regular exercise

» Managing your stress

» Treating and managing any underlying conditions that you have

» Staying fully vaccinated and boosted

Managing Long COVID Symptoms

Because no one has yet found a cure for COVID, and because Long COVID is different for everyone, managing Long COVID comes down to targeting and treating your specific symptoms and your impacted body systems. Symptoms can be mild or severe. They can be singular or multiple. COVID-19 affects many different organs and systems in the body.

In fact, no organ or system may be exempt. As researchers continue to study Long COVID, more symptoms and impacts emerge — everything from insomnia to memory loss, from aching muscles to immobility, from distortion of taste to cardiac failure. In the following sections, I describe some of the most common symptoms (but these symptoms are by no means an exhaustive list).

Symptoms of Long COVID caused by an overactive immune system — such as fatigue and joint pains — can get better with time. Symptoms caused by damage to a part of the body — such as your lungs — often won't go away, but you can improve those symptoms with good medical care.

TIP

When you're dealing with Long COVID, you may have to seek out support and information in places outside of the norm. Definitely talk to your doctor and other medical professionals about any struggles that you're having. Keep an open mind and get creative when searching for answers to what might relieve your suffering.

Fatigue

One of the most common symptoms of Long COVID is fatigue. This symptom goes beyond just feeling more tired than usual, and it lasts for an extended period of time. If you have *fatigue* from Long COVID, you may feel an intense, deep exhaustion that is constant, whether you're active or not. Even when you rest or sleep, the fatigue from Long COVID may not improve.

You may have felt fatigue before, but Long COVID fatigue can be debilitating. It often goes beyond making you just physically exhausted. You often feel totally fatigued cognitively and mentally, and you may find that you don't have the energy to function well enough to engage with your usual quality of life. Your Long COVID fatigue can sometimes be severe enough to make even simple activities — such as showering or dressing, or even just talking with someone else — feel extremely challenging.

REMEMBER

Long COVID fatigue can be very different from the normal tiredness you feel when you're sick, and it persists or recurs over an extended period, often lasting for several months after the acute phase of the infection has passed.

Your fatigue level may go up and down from day to day (or even from hour to hour), so take it slow and always listen to your body. You may also find that your fatigue develops a natural rhythm, making you less or more tired at different times of the day. If you need to accomplish a task that requires energy and you don't have help, plan to do it at your strongest time of day.

TIP

Get used to saying no! This type of fatigue is truly intense, and you can't live or work in the same way that you did before it. Set clear and firm boundaries with your employer, coworkers, family, and friends. Speak up and tell them when something is too much for you. It's okay to rest when you need to. If you want to know more about your rights at work and how to assert them legally, turn to the section later in this chapter called "Long COVID and ADA Requirements."

Respiratory and pulmonary decline

Although Long COVID can impact the entire body, it primarily affects your lungs and airway for weeks to months following your infection. Your lung function declines for one or more reasons:

>> Your original COVID-19 infection damaged your lung tissues.

>> You're experiencing a lingering inflammatory response, which can cause many of the symptoms I previously outlined, including fatigue, joint pains, brain fog, and cardiac or pulmonary problems.

This type of damage and reaction causes you to have related symptoms, which often appear as

>> **Coughing and/or chest congestion:** Can include chest pain, tightness, or pressure that accompanies your difficulties with breathing.

>> **Inability to breathe deeply and fully:** When you have this symptom, you may feel like you can never get enough oxygen, like you're always huffing and puffing.

>> **Ongoing shortness of breath:** Can occur even during light activity or while resting. The smallest activities can force you to sit down and catch your breath.

These symptoms can feel frustrating, scary, and tiring. If you experience any sort of trouble breathing, see a doctor for additional testing to find out more about what's happening. Your medical provider may investigate your condition by conducting tests such as

>> **X-rays** to look for infections.

>> **CT scans** to find out whether you have any blockages, masses, or other problems.

>> **Pulmonary function tests** that show how well you can breathe in and out and may also help to determine the cause of problem breathing.

>> **Exercise tolerance tests** that measure whether increased activity creates breathing challenges.

In good news, doctors are figuring out how to combine different treatments and therapies with much success. So, although you (rightly) may feel extremely distressed because you can't breathe properly, you have a lot of hope for relief:

>> **If you have mild or moderate respiratory decline:** Your doctor may give you breathing exercises that you can do at home.

>> **If you need more assistance:** Your doctor might start you on physical therapy, occupational therapy, or speech and language therapy.

>> **For additional relief:** Your doctor may prescribe inhalers or other medications, or if your lungs are in particularly bad shape, portable oxygen.

Cardiac decline

Another possible Long COVID effect is *cardiac decline*, which means that your heart isn't pumping as well as it should, and fluid backs up in your lungs. If your original COVID-19 infection impacted your heart muscle at all, you might develop certain effects, such as

>> Dizziness or feeling lightheaded

>> Unusual swelling in your legs, ankles, or feet

>> Chest pain

>> Heart palpitations

>> A rapid, slow, or irregular heart rate

>> Blood clots

>> Inflammation of the heart muscle (called *myocarditis*)

>> Shortness of breath

You can experience Long COVID cardiac symptoms even if your COVID-19 infection was mild, you were asymptomatic, or you have no history of cardiac problems.

If you have Long COVID cardiac symptoms, see a doctor for full testing, diagnosis, and treatment. Some tests your doctor may perform include

>> **Echocardiogram,** which shows how your blood moves through your heart.

>> **Electrocardiogram,** which can help determine whether your heart is beating in a normal, healthy rhythm and whether you have damage to your heart muscle.

>> **Cardiac stress test,** which assesses whether your heart can still function well when it's beating fast (for example, during exercise) and whether you are at risk of having a heart attack.

To treat you, your doctor may refer you to a cardiologist who can give you a plan to stay active within your limits — which helps you rebuild your heart's strength — and recommend a heart-healthy diet. They also likely help you make sure that you're managing any underlying related symptoms and conditions, such as high blood pressure; they may prescribe medications to improve heart function and control blood pressure.

If you have heart or lung problems as a result of Long COVID (or, really, anything), use a finger oximeter at home to regularly measure your oxygen saturation level. It should stay at 93 percent or higher. If at any time it dips below 93 percent, call your doctor right away or get to an emergency room.

Neurological and cognitive decline

Long COVID can affect your neurological system. You may have neurological symptoms caused by Long COVID because

>> The initial infection directly damaged your brain or nerves.

>> Your immune system responded too aggressively to the SARS-CoV-2 virus, and your nervous system is now inflamed.

The socio-emotional layer of long-term illness also complicates neurological impacts. If you're isolated or alone, or you're not as active in the world because of your illness, you can start feeling disengaged, depressed, and withdrawn. These additional experiences create a chicken-or-egg situation: You feel sad because you don't interact with anyone or get any brain stimulation, and then because you don't get any stimulation, you start to feel worse and decline further.

Neurological symptoms include

>> Brain fog (including confusion, impaired memory, loss of attention, and inability to concentrate)

>> Headaches

>> Dizziness or imbalance

>> Tingling or numbness in your extremities

REMEMBER

None of your symptoms are your fault. Help is out there, and you deserve to get it. Neurological impacts can feel especially shameful or embarrassing for many people. But this is a medical issue, just like a broken bone or a heart problem.

If you're struggling with any neurological symptoms, see your doctor for neurocognitive testing. Testing can fully evaluate you in areas of memory, focus, attention, and speech and language. After you receive a diagnosis, your doctor may offer any number of treatments or suggest at-home practices that you can take up to help you build up your neurological and cognitive functioning. These treatments and practices may include

>> Getting proper sleep

>> Working on puzzles, brain games, or any tasks that challenge you a bit mentally

>> Keeping your stress low

>> Starting talk and other therapies — such as transcranial magnetic stimulation (TMS) — or even simple physical exercise and brain teasers and puzzles that support you mentally and emotionally

>> Finding support groups or other types of groups that can get you socializing and connected

A distorted sense of smell and taste (parosmia)

Many people lose their sense of taste or smell while they're infected with COVID-19, but *parosmia*, defined as a distorted sense of smell and taste, is a whole different beast. If you experience parosmia as a result of Long COVID, you may not lose your sense of smell; instead, your sense of smell becomes severely distorted. Some smells simply smell like something they aren't, but many smells become absolutely foul and repulsive.

Scientists have yet to fully determine why COVID (and some other viruses, like the common cold) causes parosmia, but they think it relates to the original infection from the SARS-CoV-2 virus damaging the olfactory nerve cells in your nose. When your body starts generating new cells and repairing the connections between your nasal cavity and brain, something goes terribly wrong. Researchers are still trying to figure out why.

Parosmia can take a toll on you, both physically and mentally. Be aware of these factors if you're dealing with this condition:

WARNING

>> **Because smells are highly distorted, you may not be able to smell signs of danger** (such as burning food, smoke, or natural gas). If you have parosmia, make sure that all of your smoke and gas detectors are in working order and tell people to alert you if they smell something that could be dangerous.

>> **The distortion can make it impossible for you to eat without getting nauseated** because of the smell that you're perceiving. Many people who have parosmia struggle to eat enough, and they experience massive weight loss. If you have parosmia long enough, you may also find yourself becoming depressed, feeling hopeless and distressed that you can never enjoy eating again.

REMEMBER

>> **Parosmia is usually temporary, although it can persist for a long time** — for more than a year, in some cases. (And worse than that, some people seemingly have permanent parosmia.) It can take a long time to get your normal sense of smell back, but most patients end up recovering it fully — some good news about this condition.

Make an appointment with your doctor if you're struggling with parosmia. They can evaluate the information you give them about your health history, recent infections, current medications, and smoking status. They may also present different scents for you to smell and identify so that they can get an idea of how much you're struggling. They may also do an MRI, CT scan, or biopsy of your sinus tissue to look for areas of abnormal inactivity, damaged tissue, or cancerous tissue.

Although you can find living with parosmia challenging, and we doctors don't currently have a cure (other than time leading to healing, in most cases), if you get diagnosed with it, some treatments can ease your suffering, including

>> Medications

>> Olfactory/smell training where you use a kit to sniff the same four or five scents every day for several days while concentrating on telling yourself what the scents are

>> Surgery on damaged sensory receptors in the nose

Digestive issues

As a result of COVID-19, you may have serious digestive problems, some of which can lead to marked weight loss for some people. Scientists still don't know why COVID causes digestive problems, but they have several theories, such as

>> The virus directly infects cells in the gastrointestinal tract, causing inflammation and symptoms.

>> The virus disrupts the gut microbiome.

>> The immune system overreacts to the virus, leading to inflammation in the gut.

The specific symptoms that you may have include

>> Constant nausea

>> Vomiting

>> Diarrhea

>> Abdominal pain

>> Gastroesophageal reflux disease (GERD)

>> Heartburn

>> Regurgitation

>> Loss of appetite

See your doctor if you have these ongoing symptoms, and they can help you come up with a plan to manage them so that you can live more comfortably and safely. They may recommend

>> **Modifying your diet** to make it low in fat and processed foods, and high in whole grains and other plant-based food. This type of diet (although beneficial for anyone's health) can be extra helpful in keeping the digestive system healthy for people suffering from COVID-related GI issues.

>> **Taking medication** to treat specific symptoms.

>> **Drinking more water,** up to 3-4 liters per day. Staying properly hydrated keeps food moving through your digestive system well.

>> **Adding probiotics** into your daily routine by taking them in pill, powder, or even yogurt form. Probiotics lower the amount of bad bacteria in your gut and add in good bacteria. If you are eating yogurt for this purpose, be sure that it includes live bacterial cultures.

TIP

If you don't want this condition to isolate you, it doesn't have to! You can still go out and about. But until you find a plan that helps you keep food down and in, you may need to make sure you always have access to a bathroom. Plan ahead and maybe confide in a loved one who can assist you in scouting out the bathroom location, and helping if you have a bathroom emergency.

Joint and muscle pain (arthralgia and myalgia)

Like all Long COVID symptoms, scientists still don't know for sure what causes joint and muscle pain (called *arthralgia* and *myalgia*), but the prevailing theory is similar to some others. Many researchers believe this pain comes as a result of an over-active immune response to the initial infection and the associated ongoing inflammation.

If you have joint and muscle pain from COVID-19, you might feel

>> Constant aches
>> Sharp pain
>> Stiffness
>> Tingling
>> Weakness
>> A heavy feeling

You may experience any of these symptoms in one or more muscles or joints, although you're most likely to feel it in your limbs, back, and neck. The pain might be persistent, or it might come and go.

See a doctor if these symptoms persist or are severe enough that they interfere with your daily life. Your doctor may take your medical history, give you a physical exam, and maybe even do an MRI or CT scan to get a closer look at your brain or areas causing pain. They'll make sure that your pain doesn't stem from an underlying condition, such as a cancerous tumor, rather than COVID.

To manage these symptoms, you can

>> Get plenty of rest.
>> Exercise lightly under your doctor's guidance to improve your flexibility and strength.
>> Take over-the-counter pain relievers, such as ibuprofen, naproxen, or acetaminophen. The combination of ibuprofen or naproxen plus acetaminophen can be especially effective.
>> Go to physical therapy if your doctor prescribes it.
>> Keep stress low and do things that keep you relaxed.
>> Pace yourself when you're active, even if you're just doing chores around the house.
>> Apply ice or heat to the painful muscles or joints, as needed.

Maintaining Your Health and Keeping Up Your Spirits

You may feel overwhelmed navigating the uncertain waters of Long COVID, but mindset and self-care can powerfully and positively impact your recovery. Taking care of your mental health is just as important as taking care of your physical health. Your mind, body, and spirit are all connected.

The key to caring for your mental health is to embrace what you love and try to work those items and activities into a manageable daily routine. You might enjoy something such as reading or listening to audiobooks, hearing the songs of birds outside your window or from your front porch, or visiting with loved ones.

TIP

Resist the urge to overload yourself with activities. Start small and simple so that you don't get too overwhelmed or tired. Choose one or two things at first to add into your days to spice them up.

Allowing yourself to indulge in these pleasures at a reasonable pace gets your mind off of your bothersome Long COVID symptoms and reminds you that you still have a world and life out there, beyond and in spite of COVID. Keep these suggestions in mind:

>> **Get outside of your house if you're able.** Even if you don't have the energy to be very active for very long, just go for a walk around the block or simply sit outside in your garden. The fresh air and sun are good for your body, and the stimulation is good for your brain. Connecting with nature and the outside world can be key to beating feelings of isolation.

TIP

>> **Ask loved ones to help.** If you don't know what to do to add daily activities on your own, ask your loved ones for ideas. If you need extra support executing your vision, have them come along. You'll both feel better for it.

>> **Try reaching out to more people.** Whether they're your friends and family or even support groups, engage with others for extra support. You can access support groups and communities online to stay connected with others. Building a network of different activities, interests, and people can help you get through the different types of low points that you may experience.

>> **Look into therapy with a licensed professional.** And if building a network and activities with your family and friends doesn't provide enough support to feel better, you may benefit from seeking advice from a licensed professional. You can go to sessions in person, do it over the phone, or even use telehealth apps that have secure videoconferencing and chatting features.

Give yourself hope — but also, grace. Having bad days — and feeling frustrated, scared, or upset — is normal. Be patient with yourself. Recovery from Long COVID and a return to a feeling of wellness takes time, and that's okay. Celebrate your small victories and don't be too hard on yourself on the tough days. You're not alone in this journey.

Knowing how long Long COVID might last

Scientists don't yet have a definitive answer, but most Long COVID symptoms last at least three months and improve within a year. That said, some people do have symptoms more than a year after their COVID-19 infection.

You can't know how long your particular symptoms will last. You have to just take it one day at a time and try not to get too discouraged.

Going back to health basics

When you're battling Long COVID, do everything you can to keep the rest of your health in order. Eat right (I know this can be a major challenge if your Long COVID symptom is parosmia, discussed in the section "Parosmia," earlier in the chapter), sleep well (challenging if you now have insomnia), and exercise regularly (difficult if you're still struggling with respiratory, circulatory, or cardiac issues).

But as much as you can, follow these general guidelines to give your body the best chance in the fight against Long COVID:

>> **Eat a well-balanced diet** to keep your immune system strong and give yourself energy to battle fatigue. Include plenty of fruits, vegetables, lean proteins, and whole grains in your meals, and stay well hydrated. Water is the key to all life!

If you don't have much of an appetite, or your disordered taste or smell is throwing you off, eat small, frequent snacks and meals of the foods that you can stomach, even if it's not perfectly balanced. A bite of anything is better than a bite of nothing. If you have the option of no calories at all or imperfect calories, eat imperfect calories. Consult your healthcare provider if you're really struggling with eating.

>> **Stay active.** Do physical activity every day at whatever level you can to help rebuild your strength and stamina, and also boost your mood. Start slowly with short walks or stretching, and gradually increase the challenge while you get stronger. Don't push yourself too much, though. Listen to your body, and rest when you need to.

If you want some extra guidance, talk to your doctor or other medical professional who has experience with Long COVID patients. Many healthcare facilities now have programs that specialize in the care of people with Long COVID. If exercise really gets you going, come up with some workout plans and goals.

>> **Rest!** Sleep and rest as much as your body is telling you to — that's how you heal.

>> **Celebrate your improvements and accomplishments,** no matter how small! For example, treat yourself to an ice-cream cone when you clean the house!

Don't let lingering symptoms get you down

If you have Long COVID, the first six months can be the most difficult because you can have very severe symptoms with barely noticeable improvement — but you have to hang in there. Everyone has a different Long COVID experience, of course, but by around the year or year-and-a-half mark, many patients notice distinct improvement.

REMEMBER

If you have symptoms that don't improve, you can feel hopeless. But thousands (if not millions) of people who have Long COVID are powering through, so you are not alone. And because it affects so many people, researchers are very motivated to continue their work to ease the symptoms and treat Long COVID.

To prevent themselves from getting too depressed or feeling defeated by Long COVID, some people:

>> Focus their energy on tracking their symptoms and noting when they see improvement to help them stay optimistic

>> Distract themselves with socialization or taking up a new hobby

>> Read about others' success stories online (try typing "Long COVID success stories" into the search bar)

Try to keep putting one foot in front of the other. You *can* come out on the other end of this diagnosis.

Long-COVID and ADA Requirements

The Americans with Disabilities Act (ADA) protects people who have disabilities, including certain people who have had COVID-19. Under the ADA, an individual is considered to have a disability if they

>> Have a physical or mental impairment that substantially limits one or more major life activities

>> Have a medical record of such an impairment

>> Are regarded as having such an impairment by a doctor

Depending on how long and severe your COVID symptoms were, whether you still have them, and how they impact your current daily life, you may qualify for benefits and protections, such as

>> **Reasonable accommodation:** Your employer must provide you with reasonable accommodations, as long as those accommodations don't cause undue hardship for the business. If you suffer from Long COVID, you might need flexible work hours or the ability to work remotely, for example.

>> **Non-discrimination:** Your potential or actual employer can't pass you over for hiring, promotions, or other benefits and opportunities based solely on your COVID-19 status.

>> **Confidentiality of medical information:** Your employer must keep your medical information confidential and stored separately from general personnel files, which includes your COVID-19 status and any related conditions.

>> **Public accommodations and services:** You must have equal access to public accommodations and services. For example, if you now need a service animal because of Long COVID symptoms, or you need information read to you because your Long COVID symptoms make you too fatigued when reading, your employer must allow and provide the items you need.

REMEMBER

The ADA is a federal act, but laws that govern disability rights vary from state to state, so always check your specific location's details. You may have additional protections under your state law.

If you need protection under the ADA because of your Long COVID, see a lawyer or other legal professional who specializes in ADA and disability law.

3

Accepting COVID-19 Is Here to Stay

IN THIS CHAPTER

» **Evaluating the state of COVID-19 beyond the 2020 pandemic**

» **Keeping tabs on the virus variants**

» **Funding ongoing research, treatment, and testing**

» **Shoring up healthcare for long-term needs and future pandemics**

» **Staying alert against misinformation**

Chapter **10**
Looking Ahead

O n May 5, 2023, the World Health Organization (WHO) declared that COVID-19 no longer qualified as a global health emergency — but you can't totally forget about it. People will remain susceptible to catching SARS-CoV-2 and getting sick with COVID-19 for years to come (possibly for the rest of their lives, in the same way that you can catch influenza and other common viruses year after year).

None of us can predict the future, but the medical community is using what it has figured out so far about COVID-19 to make its best guesses about how to keep the disease at bay. From permanent public health policies and effective information campaigns, to ongoing research into vaccines and variants, the lasting impact of COVID-19 is everywhere, even if people don't feel or see it as obviously as they did at the height of the pandemic.

In this chapter, I give you an overview of how the world is dealing with the virus beyond the pandemic, and I also share insights about what people can possibly expect from COVID-19 in the years to come.

Taking In the General Outlook

The influence of COVID-19 looks significantly different now than it did when it first took hold of the world in 2020: The world is thankfully no longer in a pandemic at the time I'm writing this book. Doctors and the general public know much more about how the SARS-CoV-2 virus spreads and how to control it. And you can now find vaccines (which can help prevent you from contracting the disease and lessen the severity of symptoms if you do contract it) widely available.

Public health experts now see COVID-19 as an *endemic disease*, which means it's present in the population at all times, but generally at low levels — just like influenza. Public health officials, the medical community, and people around the world have come together to dramatically reduce COVID-19's global severity and death rate through widespread testing and treatment, and high global vaccination rates.

REMEMBER

But don't let the strides that the world has made give you a false sense of security. COVID-19 will always be a clear and present concern to some degree because variants of the virus continue to pop up (although we in the medical community can often knock them down just as quickly, thanks to mRNA vaccines, which you can read about in Chapter 2). Also, many people must manage Long COVID symptoms. (I talk about Long COVID in Chapter 9.)

Although scientists may never be able to completely eradicate the virus, medical professionals, public health agencies, and the public are keeping COVID-19 under control. Measures such as ensuring everyone around the world has access to vaccines, continuing to improve and evolve treatment methods, and fine-tuning public health responses work not only for COVID-19, but also for possible future pandemics.

Examining future developments in the U.S.

Overall, the U.S. is managing COVID-19 better at the time this book is going to press than it did during the pandemic. Few people are dying from COVID-19 now that the pandemic is over. A big reason for this significant drop in mortality involves the fact that about 70 to 80 percent of the population is fully vaccinated against COVID-19.

WARNING

Far fewer people have received the Omicron variant booster vaccine, and if more people don't keep up with boosters when they become available, COVID-19 may make a resurgence.

Also, Long COVID still affects millions of people's ability to return to work and lead healthy lives. In June 2022, the U.S. Census Bureau asked questions about Long COVID in its Household Pulse Survey, the answers to which revealed these staggering statistics:

>> Sixteen million Americans between the ages of 18 and 65 have Long COVID.

>> Two to four million people who have Long COVID are out of work because of it.

>> Lost annual wages for people who have Long COVID fall somewhere in the range of $170 to $230 billion.

REMEMBER

As outlined in a report from Brookings Metro (a research program through the nonprofit Brookings Institute that advocates for public policy changes and practical solutions to systemic problems) published in January 2022, Long COVID may be the biggest threat to the U.S. public's long-term public health and economy.

Despite the U.S.'s high vaccination rate, scientists still don't have a good treatment for Long COVID. For the U.S. to weather Long COVID within its population, these groups within the country need to continue to improve their standard operating procedures in several ways:

>> **Employers:** Provide extended sick leave and workplace accommodations that meet the needs of those who have symptoms.

>> **Researchers:** Develop even more effective prevention and treatment options.

>> **The federal government:** Expand disability benefits and increase funding and oversight of Long COVID studies.

Assessing COVID-19 preparedness in other countries

Other developed countries (such as the U.K.) face many — if not all — of the same Long COVID challenges that the U.S. does. And so, these countries need to keep the same emphasis on maintaining a vaccinated population and providing research and funding to counteract the effects of Long COVID that I discuss in the preceding section in relation to the U.S.

Many vulnerable, developing, and low-income countries (for example, Haiti, at the time of this writing) are still struggling to monitor and report COVID-19 cases, as well as to treat them. Here are some of the challenges that these countries face:

>> **Inadequate infrastructure:** Because they lack the means to dispense large supplies of COVID-19 vaccines quickly, these countries can't accept all types of vaccines. They need vaccines that have longer shelf lives of nine or more months, as opposed to the typical six months, as well as vaccines that have less rigorous storage requirements (for example, perhaps the vaccines don't need to be stored in a freezer).

>> **A struggle to keep everyone fully vaccinated against COVID-19:** Low-income countries may have to decline vaccine shipments that don't meet the requirements demanded by their lack of infrastructure and resources. As a result, their populations can fall behind on maintaining vaccinated status.

REMEMBER

On a positive note, some pharmaceutical companies are providing low-income countries with supplies of their COVID-19 antiviral medications at low or no cost.

>> **Secondary impacts on economic, food, nutrition, and education factors:** Losing so much income and education during the global COVID-19 shutdown has been especially devastating for low-income countries. For example, in July 2023, the State of Food Security and Nutrition in the World (SOFI) 2023, published by the Food and Agriculture Organization (FAO), showed that "more than 3.1 billion people worldwide couldn't afford a healthy diet in 2021. . .an increase of 134 million people compared to 2019 before the onset of the COVID-19 pandemic."

WARNING

The Bill and Melinda Gates Foundation suggests the COVID-19 pandemic caused "a setback of about 25 years in about 25 weeks" with regard to health, economy, and overall global development, and that extreme poverty will rise globally by up to 150 million more people affected.

Monitoring the Mutations

In June 2020, the World Health Organization (WHO) started the Virus Evolution Working Group (later renamed Technical Advisory Group on SARS-CoV-2 Virus Evolution) to monitor SARS-CoV-2 variants. Since then, this group has created a labeling and prioritization system to let the medical community around the world know which variants pose more of a threat to public health than others. The WHO's work with this system has helped them rapidly share their risk assessments with the world so that public health agencies around the globe can respond quickly and effectively.

WHO uses their system to monitor SARS-CoV-2 not only in humans, but also in animal populations. Continuing to monitor relevant species (for example, bats) closely for this virus can tell scientists when new variants emerge before they affect humans — a key element in managing and reducing mutations around the world.

WHO continues to update its tracking system and working definitions for variants of concern, variants of interest, and variants under monitoring, with the most recent update being March 2023, as of this book's writing.

Funding for Future Developments

While the pandemic has slowed, funding for COVID-19 research and treatment has, too. However, if governments and public health agencies in the U.S. and around the world want to keep their populations healthy, they need to continue to fund research, testing, and treatment — and more than that, improve oversight of the funding they do give. See the sidebar "What is NIH doing?" for an example of the need for funding oversight.

For research and treatment

During the pandemic, the U.S. and other governments offered plentiful funding for COVID-19 research in order to help medical researchers determine the cause, treatment, and prevention of COVID-19. Post-pandemic funding for COVID-19 research is a different story.

WHAT IS NIH DOING?

The National Institutes of Health (NIH) received $1 billion from Congress in 2020 to research Long COVID, but while I write this book, they've produced no results. They haven't registered any patients for trials yet — which may actually have a silver lining to it, considering some health experts say the trial related to exercise may cause more damage to patients than provide help. They've mostly studied patients by observation, but they haven't published any findings yet.

Inexplicably, no one has pressed the NIH for accountability. However, when the delinquency of the NIH came to light in the media — as in an article by Rachel Cohrs that published in *STAT* in March 2022 — other government agencies stepped up to fill the need. For example, the U.S. Department of Health and Human Services (HHS) and the Agency for Healthcare Research and Quality (AHRQ) worked together to start a $9 million annual initiative for funding Long COVID clinical trials.

Despite the fact that Long COVID threatens long-term public health, now that the pandemic is over, government funding for COVID-19 research has declined. In response, several private foundations around the world have emerged to offer funding, such as

>> Long COVID Research Initiative (U.S.)

>> Solve Long COVID Initiative (U.S.)

>> Stichting Long COVID (Netherlands)

For testing

Some government agencies no longer fund COVID-19 testing, although some private insurance companies and nonprofit agencies may provide you with free tests if you need them.

TIP

If you need COVID-19 testing and can't afford to purchase tests, try visiting

>> Your local public health department

>> Community health clinics and organizations

>> Pharmacies

Not all of these entities offer free testing or test kits, but they give you a good place to start. Visit their websites or call them before your visit to see whether they offer free testing or kits. Also, see Chapter 7 for more about testing for COVID-19.

Ensuring Essential Healthcare Services

The pandemic taught the world that all nations need robust healthcare systems, not only so that patients can receive the care they need, but also to slow and potentially end the spread of deadly disease. Since the pandemic, countries across the globe have

>> **Expanded telehealth,** providing prompt healthcare to patients in remote locations, patients who are too sick to travel to a facility, or patients who have limited or no mobility.

>> **Implemented strategies to improve the experience of healthcare workers,** such as cross-training, mental health support, and initiatives to attract more people to the field.

>> **Improved supply chain management** to make sure that they have enough PPE and other vital supplies on hand, as well as effective and efficient ways to get more supplies before levels get dangerously low.

Preserving Stability and Preventing Outbreaks

To maintain our current stability and prevent future outbreaks of COVID-19, governments, health agencies, and individuals can work together in many ways. You (and everyone you know) can follow these tips to keep COVID-19 under control in your own life:

>> **Stay alert and aware:** Even though, at the time of this writing, COVID-19 isn't as big of a threat as it was during the height of the pandemic, it's still an active virus. If people let down their guard too much — for example, by not isolating when they have symptoms — COVID-19 might make a resurgence.

>> **Get vaccinated:** Stay current with your COVID-19 vaccines. Get boosted when and if you should, as indicated by the U.S. CDC or your government's health agency. The more people who get vaccinated, the more effectively we can reduce the severity of the disease and reduce the spread of COVID-19.

>> **Practice good health and hygiene:** Wear a mask in risky settings (such as when you're indoors and in contact with people who have symptoms), wash your hands well and often, and practice social distancing, particularly in crowded and poorly ventilated spaces.

Beyond the individual, governments, and public health organizations need to take steps to help prevent another pandemic by

>> **Monitoring public health and responding rapidly:** Continue to watch for new variants, conduct widespread and accessible testing, and coordinate contact tracing and isolation when needed — and before the virus reaches pandemic levels again.

>> **Creating and maintaining robust healthcare systems:** Ensure that nations have ample hospital capacity, the right type and amount of necessary equipment, and well-trained healthcare workers in place across facilities to provide effective treatments and to manage those who do get infected, while still caring for non-COVID-19 patients.

>> **Providing clear, accurate communication (and following it):** Provide clear, consistent, and transparent messaging to build public trust and ensure that people understand how to protect themselves and their communities.

TIP

As citizens, all people should follow the guidance from these reputable sources and share only science-backed information. For more on the impact of misinformation, see the following section.

>> **Cooperating globally:** Seeing as how national borders don't stop viruses, governments across the world need to share information in a timely way, as well as resources, including making sure that all countries have access to affordable vaccines for their citizens. If one country experiences a fresh outbreak, the whole world is at risk.

>> **Preparing for future outbreaks:** Another outbreak *will* happen at some point. Governments and public health agencies need to not only develop plans for future response, but also continue to provide funding and research, and maintain reserves of essential supplies so that they can respond quickly at the first signs of an outbreak.

REMEMBER

All people play a part in keeping COVID-19 at bay. If the pandemic taught us nothing else, we hopefully now realize that all citizens (regardless of country) truly are members of a global community. What happens to one person or country happens to us all.

Mitigating Misinformation

Misinformation always poses a threat to public health and can erode trust in the scientific community and the scientific process. The public health community continues to battle misinformation, even today. During the height of the pandemic, many news outlets and even social media platforms worked together to crack down on false posts, articles, and other communications. But despite these best efforts, misinformation found its way to the public.

And after the WHO declared COVID-19 no longer a global health emergency, many platforms (for example, Meta and X) relaxed their misinformation policies and practices, causing some health experts to worry about an increase in false information circulating as fact again.

Feeling the effects of past misinformation

People around the world are still recovering from the falsehoods about the SARS-CoV-2 virus; its origins; and the effectiveness of masks, social distancing, and vaccines that many people (and even some media outlets and political leaders) spread in the early days of the pandemic.

REMEMBER

Because of this conflicting guidance and early misinformation, many people still hesitate or refuse to follow public health guidelines or get vaccinated. This lack of compliance with preventative measures means that COVID-19 will continue to spread to some degree. Beyond affecting individual behaviors, misinformation continues to divide people and lead them to mistrust public health institutions.

Battling misinformation going forward

WARNING

If citizens and media organizations become too lax with efforts to fight misinformation, the world could find itself experiencing an increase in COVID-19 cases and deaths once again.

While the world moves beyond the COVID-19 pandemic, public health organizations, governments, and the general public always have to actively battle misinformation to help keep the virus at bay. Individuals, governments, health organizations, and social media platforms must remain committed to sharing accurate, science-based information to keep our global society healthy.

TIP

To do your part, make sure that you fact-check any information about COVID-19 before you share it. Ensure that you're sharing from a reputable and science-based source.

IN THIS CHAPTER

» **Knowing how to prevent spreading COVID-19 at work**

» **Staying safe around others who are sick**

» **Taking steps after you've been exposed to COVID-19**

» **Acting fast if you have symptoms at work**

» **Evaluating when you can go back to work**

Chapter **11**

Staying Safe When Working Outside Your Home

I f you work outside your home and have to spend time around other employees or members of the public regularly, you most likely have a greater risk of contracting or spreading COVID-19 than do people who work from home.

Here's the good news: Since the pandemic of 2020, many companies have rewritten their workplace sick leave and hygiene policies in order to accommodate for people who are impacted by COVID-19 — and need time off to go to the doctor — or who need to work remotely to prevent spreading the virus. Businesses also may have implemented wellness practices, such as messaging out "stay home if you have symptoms," to reduce the likelihood of staff members becoming sick with and transmitting COVID-19 to each other.

But here's the bad news: Not all companies commit equally to maintaining the ongoing health and safety of their employees.

And of course, different workplaces have different levels of inherent risk, based simply on their industry (for example, doctors and nurses who see sick patients all day every day have a higher risk of contracting COVID-19 than accountants who sit in their private offices most of the time).

In this chapter, I focus on workers outside of the healthcare industry. This chapter can help non-healthcare employees — such as office, retail, factory, or food industry workers — stay as safe and healthy as possible at work.

An Ounce of Prevention Is Worth a Pound of Cure

Prevention, prevention, prevention. Take steps to prevent yourself from contracting or spreading COVID-19. Preventing the disease is considerably easier and less stressful than treating it. Keeping your vaccine current and washing your hands regularly is much simpler (and easier on your body) than experiencing the illness and going through treatment, which can be long and daunting, especially in severe cases. (Chapter 8 describes treatments for COVID-19.)

REMEMBER

Even if you get a mild case of COVID-19, it can take a potentially harsh and long-lasting physical toll on you. And isolating and worrying about transmitting the virus to loved ones can cause emotional distress that far outweighs the minor inconveniences of using preventive measures.

While in the workplace, you can take three major prevention steps to help keep COVID-19 at bay: Use personal protective equipment (PPE), maintain good hygiene, and ensure proper ventilation.

Using PPE

One way to prevent spreading or catching COVID-19 at work involves using *personal protective equipment* (PPE), such as masks, gloves, and other items designed to shield against infection. Not all industries carry the same risk, so you may not need to use every item available.

If your workplace requires you to interact with other people, food, or other consumables in a close setting, to protect yourself and others from infection, adopt these practices:

>> Wear a mask, gloves, and apron while preparing or serving consumables.

>> Wear a mask while interacting with other people at close proximity, such as at the front counter, fitting areas in retail stores, or hair salons.

>> Use face shields or protective clothing for added protection if you're in extra-tight or risky quarters, such as working on an assembly line in a factory.

WARNING

Don't rely only on plexiglass barriers. Medical researchers haven't found evidence that they provide a barrier from germs. Instead, they may impede air circulation, meaning if someone on one side of the barrier has COVID-19 and expels droplets into the air, those droplets have a greater chance of landing on others who are on the same side of the barrier. For example, if a shared checkout stand includes a shield between the employees and customers, and one coworker contaminates the air, they may infect coworkers who share their workspace. See Chapter 5 for more information about how COVID-19 is transmitted.

If your workplace hasn't provided you with PPE and health and safety training to reduce or prevent COVID-19, contact your HR department to find out what help and information they offer and how you can access it.

Maintaining good hygiene

In the workplace, designing and implementing a quality hygiene policy and procedure is key to preventing the spread of COVID-19. You and your coworkers should

>> **Wash your hands frequently and thoroughly** with soap and water for at least 20 seconds, especially after touching common surfaces, before and after breaks, before and after touching food and using shared equipment, and after using the restroom.

TIP

You can use hand sanitizer that contains at least 60 percent alcohol if you don't have access to soap and water.

» **Cover your mouth and nose** with a tissue or the inside of your elbow when coughing or sneezing. Throw away used tissues and wash your hands immediately afterwards. Check out Chapter 5 if you want to read more about how you transmit COVID-19.

» **Avoid sharing personal items** — especially items such as mobile phones, earbuds, or makeup — that come into regular contact with your face.

» **Stay home if you feel sick.** Also, test yourself for COVID-19 right away so that, if you test positive, you can inform any coworkers you've recently been in contact with immediately. See Chapter 7 for information on COVID-19 testing.

Although the world has weathered the 2020 COVID-19 pandemic, it never hurts to practice good hygiene in the workplace, even if some of your coworkers look at you funny for being extra cautious. In addition to lessening the chance of getting COVID, these measures can protect you and your coworkers from many other infections, such as a common cold and influenza.

Ensuring proper ventilation

Maintaining good ventilation in the workplace is one of the most powerful ways to minimize the spread of COVID-19 because it keeps air and any particles in the air moving, rather than settling on (and in) you.

REMEMBER

As an employee, you may not have control over big things — for example, what kind of heating, ventilation, and air conditioning (HVAC) system your workplace has installed — but you can do small things to improve air quality that can add up, such as

» **Keeping your windows and doors open.** Opening up your work area improves the flow of air and allows potentially harmful air components to disperse.

» **Using personal or room HEPA air filters** in your office or workspace, if allowed.

» **Asking management to have the company's HVAC system serviced regularly.** Also, ask whether your employer can have the HVAC servicers increase the amount of outdoor air that the system brings in, versus re-circulating indoor air.

» **Holding meetings outdoors or remotely** when possible. And if you do have to gather in person and indoors, keep the meeting's attendance small.

If you want to dive further into the ins and outs of ventilation, check out Chapter 6.

TIP

If you're in a position to make decisions about operations and budgets, spend the money on a quality HVAC system and maintenance. Although you may have a steep upfront cost, good ventilation is an invaluable investment because it helps everyone stay healthy, keeping employee (and customer) absenteeism low in the long run.

Watching Out for Others with COVID-19 Symptoms

If you're in contact with a coworker or customer you think might be sick, don't ignore it or brush it off. You don't have to be rude or make a big scene about their perceived condition, but you can do a few things to help them, and to make sure that you and other healthy coworkers and customers stay that way. See Chapter 5 for a description of COVID-19 symptoms.

For a coworker who shows symptoms

If you observe that a coworker has possible COVID-19 symptoms, ask them to isolate in a closed room or wear a mask until you can get in touch with a supervisor who can facilitate sending them home so that they don't spread germs to others (remember to communicate using the proper chain of command for your company).

Supervisors are legally allowed to ask employees if they have COVID-19 symptoms, but they must walk a fine line between keeping their workplaces safe and adhering to federal guidelines about disclosing employees' private health information. Don't expect managers to share details of another employee's health in a company-wide email, but passing along your observations about possible COVID-19 symptoms could help managers act in the interest of all employees' safety.

TIP

If the employee that you suspect might have COVID-19 remains at work for some reason, definitely maintain your distance and put on a mask if you can. You might even consider going home early or working remotely at another location for the rest of the day, again, if you can.

For a customer who shows symptoms

If you notice a customer who has potential COVID-19 symptoms, talk with your supervisor about appropriate steps that you can take to keep yourself safe. Depending on your company policy, you may or may not be able to ask the customer to leave. But you can definitely put on a mask and keep your distance from that customer, if nothing else.

Responding to Exposure

Not all COVID-19 exposure is the same. When you've been in contact with someone who has COVID-19, consider different risk factors and your current symptom status to respond appropriately.

Determining the risk factors

Some exposures to COVID-19 pose a higher risk than others. Logically, a high-risk exposure gives you a higher chance of contracting COVID-19 than does a low-risk exposure. In a work-place environment, you do have risk of being exposed by another person — either a coworker or a customer.

To determine the riskiness of your exposure from another person, see Table 11-1 for a rundown of the factors that impact the risk of transmission of the COVID-19 virus.

If you find out that you were in a situation where the transmission risk from a COVID-19–infected person was high, err on the side of caution. Isolate, monitor yourself for symptoms, and test yourself right away (see Chapter 7). Don't skip any steps or cut corners.

TABLE 11-1 **Risk of Exposure to COVID-19**

Factor	Situation	Risk of Transmitting or Contracting
Vaccination Status	Both people are vaccinated	Low
	One person is vaccinated, but the other person isn't	Higher (though less of a chance of transmission)
	Neither person is vaccinated	Much higher
Length of Exposure	2-minute chat at someone's desk	Low
	Talking while on a 15-minute break	Higher
Level of Activity	Normal talking	Low
	Coughing, singing, or shouting	Higher
Symptoms	Visible symptoms	Higher
	No visible symptoms	Low
Masking Status	Both people wearing masks	Low
	One person wearing a mask	Higher
	Neither person wearing a mask	Much higher
Location	Outdoors	Low
	Inside with good ventilation	Higher
	Inside with poor ventilation	Much higher
Social Distance	Sitting apart or separated by a barrier	Low
	Close together or touching	Higher

Watching for symptoms and responding

After coming into contact with someone at work who has symptoms of or tests positive for COVID-19, monitor yourself for symptoms of COVID-19, such as

» Fever

» Cough

» Loss of taste or smell

» Difficulty breathing

» Body aches

» Fatigue

If you need help figuring out if your symptoms are actually COVID-19 symptoms or just symptoms of a cold or the flu, check out Chapter 5 for information that outlines the differences between the three so that you can get a good idea of whether you should test yourself for COVID-19.

REMEMBER

Your symptoms can appear anytime within 2 to 14 days after exposure.

Even if you don't know that you've been exposed to COVID-19 at work, any time you get sick, remain cognizant of COVID-19. Don't assume that what you have is a cold and go into work anyway. Keep in mind that your illness could be COVID-19 and take the right steps to keep yourself and others at work safe:

» **If you're asymptomatic after a known exposure,** you can still go to work, but you need to wear a mask for 10 days. Test yourself for the COVID-19 virus on Day 5 after the exposure. (See Chapter 7 for information on testing.) Once you have your results, you can act accordingly.

   • *If you test negative,* go to work and go about your normal routine (just keep that mask on for 10 days).

   • *If you test positive,* isolate immediately, as I outline in the section "Isolating yourself," later in this chapter.

WARNING

If you take a test earlier than Day 5 after exposure, you may get a false negative result because, even if you do have SARS-CoV-2, your body may not have enough of the virus built up yet for tests to detect it. By Day 5, rapid antigen and PCR tests can usually detect your viral load.

» **If you're symptomatic,** isolate and test for the virus immediately and follow the guidance in the following section.

TIP

If you're using at-home COVID-19 tests, check the kits for an expiration date to make sure they're still good to use. If you have any doubts about the quality of your tests, you may want to test several times. For all of the details on how to get or take a test, see Chapter 7.

Responding to Symptoms While at Work

If you come down with symptoms such as fever, cough, loss of taste or smell, or any other COVID-19 symptoms while you're at work (see Chapter 5 for a full list), act quickly and decisively so that you can get better fast and prevent yourself from potentially spreading the virus to others.

Isolating yourself

Immediately isolate in a closed-off room or area away from other people and ask a coworker to inform your supervisor that you're concerned about the appearance of potential COVID-19 symptoms. If your company provides testing and follow up, your supervisor may guide you through that process. If not, they may simply send you home. After your supervisor releases you to go home, stay home, seek medical attention, and get tested immediately. See Chapter 7 for more information on how to quarantine after you get home and other tips for isolation.

WARNING

Some people try to tough it out and work through sickness, no matter what illness they have, but in the case of COVID-19, *don't do it.* You not only endanger your recovery, but also put others at risk of contracting the virus. Even if you don't have COVID, you could have other infections such as the flu, which can make others sick.

Reporting to your supervisor

When you tell your supervisor that you have symptoms, report the information according to your company's sick policy. Let them know that you have COVID-19 symptoms and that you plan to stay home until the symptoms improve.

If you're at home when you develop COVID-19 symptoms and have to call in sick, keep your message simple. You don't have to apologize, offer to work remotely, or give more details than necessary.

Returning to Work: The Criteria

Here's how and when you can get back to work after you've recovered from COVID-19 or after you've been exposed to it but show no signs of infection for five days.

REMEMBER

Don't return to work if you don't feel well enough to do so, even if your boss, coworkers, or others pressure you. Your health (and the health of others!) is more important than work.

After you recover

If you have COVID-19, stay home for at least five full days from the start of symptoms. (Day 1 is the first full day after symptoms begin.)

After five days, if you're fever-free for 24 hours (without using medication) and your symptoms are improving, you can go back to work without serious risk of infecting coworkers or patrons.

REMEMBER

Wear a mask through Day 10 because you can transmit COVID-19 up to 10 days after you were exposed.

If you're not improving yet after five days, continue to stay home. Wait until you meet the criteria to return.

After you were exposed but didn't get sick

If you were exposed to COVID-19 but aren't showing symptoms, you can still go to work — while wearing a mask until Day 10. Test yourself for COVID-19 on Day 5. If the test gives you a negative result, you can keep going to work masked until Day 10. After Day 10, you can remove the mask.

If you test positive on Day 5, isolate and follow the guidance in the section "Isolating yourself," earlier in this chapter.

4

The Part of Tens

Uncover the truth about the most common COVID-19 misinformation.

Reflect on how life has changed since the 2020 pandemic.

Leverage lessons from the 2020 pandemic to keep the world safe during future pandemics.

Chapter **12**

More than Ten COVID-19 Myths, Busted

From how the virus behaves to how to relieve your symptoms, if you catch COVID-19, misinformation and confusing ideas can make you struggle to know what to believe. What's fact? What's fiction? In matters of personal health and public safety, you need to stay updated with the correct information so that you can make decisions that benefit not just yourself, but everyone around you.

In this chapter, I bust 11 of the most common COVID-19 myths to help you stay safe and confident in the current best practices for COVID-19 as of this writing. You can access updated information — as the world's understanding of COVID-19 grows — by checking online with sources such as the World Health Organization (WHO), the U.S. Centers for Disease Control and Prevention (CDC), and your state and local health departments.

COVID-19 Is Just a Bad Cold or Flu

COVID-19 shares many symptoms with the common cold and the flu, *but it's not a cold or the flu.*

For starters, COVID-19 is caused by the SARS-CoV-2 virus, whereas colds and the flu are caused by other (typically milder) viruses. Compared to cold and flu viruses, SARS-CoV-2 is more contagious and can give people more severe respiratory illness. In some cases, SARS-CoV-2 can lead to people developing complications that require hospitalization or even cause death. These severe cases happen especially for people in high-risk groups, such as those who have underlying health conditions (such as diabetes, heart problems, or obesity) or seniors.

Although similar severe complications can sometimes arise if you have the flu, the likelihood of it happening is much smaller than with COVID-19 — and colds never cause those complications. (See Chapter 2 for more on the SARS-CoV-2 virus and Chapter 5 for a comparison of symptoms among colds, the flu, and COVID-19.)

Overall, cold viruses aren't as inherently dangerous as SARS-CoV-2; and cold viruses don't change very much, unlike SARS-CoV-2, which constantly evolves into new variants. And unlike the flu virus, SARS-CoV-2 doesn't impact just the respiratory system.

Some people who recover from an initial COVID-19 infection experience Long COVID (covered in Chapter 9), where they retain symptoms long-term or even develop new ones. These symptoms range from *parosmia* (a distorted sense of smell) or extreme and chronic fatigue, to heart palpitations, blood clots, cardiovascular disease, lung disease, and memory loss. The symptoms can last for months after the patient's recovery from the original COVID-19 infection; people don't typically experience such long-term effects after they have a cold or the flu.

COVID-19 Vaccines Are Risky

In general, *vaccines are very safe, and the vaccine for SARS-CoV-2 is no exception.*

Even though researchers worked quickly to create them and government agencies fast-tracked their authorization, COVID-19 vaccines went through all of the proper clinical trials and approval processes.

As of this writing, medical providers have given approximately 12.7 billion COVID-19 vaccines to people across 184 countries, so researchers now have the data to prove the vaccine's safety and effectiveness that they didn't at the start of the pandemic of 2020. (See Chapter 6 for a closer look at vaccines for COVID-19.)

Consider these details about COVID-19 vaccines and their side effects. The vaccines

>> **Don't damage your immune system:** If you experience side effects (although many people don't have any side effects), they're typically mild to moderate — just like with most vaccines — while your immune system figures out how to battle SARS-CoV-2. You can typically treat the side effects yourself at home with over-the-counter medication and resting until they subside within a few days.

>> **Rarely produce serious side effects:** Just like with any vaccine, you may experience serious effects from the COVID-19 vaccine, but those sorts of reactions are extremely rare. One side effect that data show can occur as a result of receiving the COVID-19 vaccine is *myocarditis,* which is the inflammation of the heart muscle that can cause chest pain, shortness of breath, and rapid or irregular heart rhythms.

The U.S. CDC data show that cases of myocarditis after getting the COVID-19 vaccine occur most frequently in adolescent and adult males under 40 years old within seven days after receiving the second dose of an mRNA COVID-19 vaccine. However, researchers have found that the SARS-CoV-2 virus causes myocarditis more frequently than the vaccine, and although most people who get myocarditis after the vaccine experience a mild case from which they recover quickly, those contracting it after COVID-19 often experience a more severe case.

>> **Occasionally trigger an allergic reaction:** Although it's unlikely to be severe, you might also experience an allergic reaction to the vaccine. But I like to remind people: You can be allergic to all kinds of things, including foods, but the risk of allergic reactions doesn't stop most of us from trying new foods!

Don't take everything you hear or read in the news for granted as truth. Sadly, not all politicians and leaders give truthful information and updates about the COVID-19 vaccine. Despite the overwhelming evidence of the safety and effectiveness of the

COVID-19 vaccine, prominent politicians and other leaders continue to spread misinformation and outright lies about made-up side effects and false data regarding effectiveness. When in doubt, the U.S. Centers for Disease Control and Prevention (CDC), your state and local health departments, and the World Health Organization (WHO) are reliable sources.

Any side effects from the vaccines are significantly less frequent and less severe than the effects of COVID-19 itself. We in the medical community know that the risk-to-benefit ratio is very much in favor of vaccination.

You Don't Need the Vaccine if You've Had COVID-19

Even if you've had COVID-19, still get the vaccine because *having COVID-19 once doesn't protect you from getting infected again.*

COVID-19 has a cumulative effect, so every time you get COVID-19, the symptoms can get worse, last longer, and lead to long-term health problems.

The following points support the argument for getting vaccinated, even if you previously had a COVID-19 infection:

>> **The effectiveness of your body's immunity that develops from an infection varies greatly among people.** Scientists have found that people who had COVID-19 have greater immunity against SARS-CoV-2 than people who only received the vaccine, but their research also shows that the level of effectiveness of *infection-acquired immunity* (the protection you get from past COVID-19 infections) varies greatly between people — meaning, you may be one of the lucky ones who gets great immunity post-infection, or you may not be.

Getting infected with SARS-CoV-2 to develop immunity is risky business because you can't predict how severe your COVID-19 will be. If you end up with serious symptoms, such as cardiac or respiratory problems, and you have to be hospitalized, you could experience complications that lead to Long COVID or even death. The risk isn't worth it when you can get a COVID-19 vaccine that the U.S. CDC and Food and Drug Administration (FDA) have proven is safe and effective.

» **Vaccinations can guard against future infection and keep the symptoms of any infection that does occur relatively mild.** If you previously had COVID-19, getting a vaccine helps keep you safe in the future. Bolstering your immune system by getting a vaccine can keep your symptoms mild and your recovery time short if you do get infected again, or it may prevent you from contracting COVID-19 altogether. Being vaccinated also makes it less likely that you transmit COVID-19 to others if you get infected. (See Chapter 6 about protecting yourself and others from COVID-19.)

Masking Doesn't Protect Against COVID-19

Masking is highly effective in slowing and preventing the transmission of COVID-19 according to public health organizations across the world, such as the World Health Organization (WHO) and the U.S. Centers for Disease Control and Prevention (CDC).

SARS-CoV-2 is an airborne virus. When people become infected with COVID-19 (or many other viruses), they emit respiratory droplets from their noses and mouths that contain the virus. After these droplets enter the air, they can infect other people. Masks, however, trap those droplets before they can go anywhere, significantly reducing how far and fast COVID-19 can spread.

Different masks provide different levels of protection, but as long as they fit properly, all masks provide some protection. If you want the best protection, wear an N95 mask (or a KN95 mask, which is similar). Surgical masks provide an only slightly lower level of protection than N95 masks, followed by tight-weave cloth masks. (Chapter 6 provides more detail on masks and masking.)

Sometimes, people think masking doesn't work because other factors cause them to transmit or catch COVID-19, even when they mask. For example

>> They remove their mask while still around infected people.

>> They touch their mask or other contaminated object or surface, and then touch their eyes, nose, or mouth without washing their hands.

>> Their mask has a gap or holes in it.

Like with any protective measure or personal protective equipment (PPE), masking alone can never prevent you from transmitting or catching COVID-19 with 100 percent efficacy. But as part of a whole system of good hygiene, wearing a mask can very effectively prevent you and others from spreading COVID-19.

REMEMBER

The mask doesn't work if you keep it in your pocket or in a drawer back home. But if you put it on, keep it on, and maintain good hygiene overall, it can effectively protect you and those around you from infection.

A Negative COVID-19 Test Means You Don't Have It

You can't always take a negative COVID-19 test at face value. *Even though you see a negative result on your COVID-19 test, you still could be infected.*

You may find yourself in one of these circumstances:

>> You don't have enough of the virus built up in your system yet for the test to detect it.

>> You didn't insert the swab far enough up your nose or circulate it enough to get a quality sample.

>> The test is expired, and the ingredients or parts have degraded over time.

To confirm that you get accurate test results from your COVID-19 testing, follow these steps:

1. **Take an at-home COVID-19 antigen test as soon as you suspect that you may be infected.**

   I talk about the types of tests and how to use them in Chapter 7.

2. **If you get a negative result on the test that you take in Step 1, test yourself again with an antigen test in 48 hours.**

The second test is especially important if you have symptoms or have come in contact with a person who has COVID-19.

TIP

Fun fact: Did you know most at-home antigen test kits include two tests for this exact situation?

3. **If you get another negative test result in Step 2, but you have COVID-19 symptoms or were exposed to COVID-19, take a PCR test.**

PCR tests are more sensitive than antigen tests and can detect a smaller amount of the virus.

REMEMBER

If you get a negative result (or two) on your antigen test — and are asymptomatic and have not been knowingly exposed to COVID-19 — you most likely don't have it.

Rubbing Alcohol and Disinfectants Cure COVID-19

WARNING

Rubbing alcohol and disinfectant aren't safe for people to inject or ingest

Both compounds kill germs on surfaces, such as tabletops and counters, but they can't treat any sort of internal infection. And if you inject or ingest these substances into your body, you could suffer from gastrointestinal distress, organ damage, coma, or even death.

As of this writing, no one has developed a cure for COVID-19, but you can treat it by using several different medications, including

>> Remdesivir (brand name Veklury)

>> Nirmatrelvir/ritonavir (brand name Paxlovid)

>> Molnupiravir (brand name Lagevrio)

>> Steroids

For more information on each of these treatments, turn to Chapter 8, where I discuss them in detail.

Rapid Tests Aren't Effective

Rapid antigen tests are very effective at giving you results in about 15 minutes, which makes them a better choice over a PCR test that may take a day or two to give you results.

Rapid antigen tests are less sensitive than PCR tests, and they need more of the virus to trigger a positive result. These characteristics make them very effective at helping you determine whether you're contagious (because if you have enough of the virus in your body that it gives you a positive rapid test, you're probably at peak transmission level).

The only drawback to using rapid antigen tests: Because they're less sensitive, you may get a negative result when you actually do have COVID-19 if you don't test during your peak infection level (about three to five days after symptoms start). But if you take a rapid antigen test during that three-to-five-day peak-infection window, you most likely get an accurate positive.

TIP

If you get a negative result from a rapid antigen test, that doesn't necessarily tell you that you're not infected. Follow up by either taking a PCR test or by doing another rapid antigen test 48 hours later. See the section "A Negative COVID-19 Test Means You Don't Have It" earlier in this chapter.

You Have to Pay for COVID-19 Tests

Even though the 2020 pandemic is over, you can still get tested for free in some places.

The U.S. Centers for Disease Control and Prevention (CDC) program called Increasing Community Access to Testing (ICATT) still offers no-cost testing for people without insurance who have symptoms of or who were exposed to COVID-19. You can visit the CDC's Search for No-Cost COVID-19 Testing page at http://testinglocator.cdc.gov to find a testing location near you. Also, many insurance plans still cover testing for COVID-19.

COVID-19 Is so Mild Now, It's Okay to Get It

Even though vaccinations against COVID-19 and treatments for the illness increase survival rates and decrease the length of infection and suffering, as compared to at the height of the pandemic in 2020, *no one can just forget about COVID-19.*

Consider other diseases that the medical community has figured out effective ways to prevent and treat, such as tuberculosis or HIV. Medical experts and public health agencies hope to remove diseases or viruses in one of two ways:

>> **Eradicate:** Remove a disease or virus across the entire globe permanently (smallpox is the only virus in history that medical science has successfully eradicated).

>> **Eliminate:** Wipe out diseases or viruses locally for long periods of time (efforts have managed to often eliminate measles and polio from regions for years).

KEEPING UP THE COVID-19 DEFENSES

Humanity can't simply ignore the ongoing threat that COVID-19 poses, even when the medical community has the disease under control. And although the lockdowns during the COVID-19 pandemic contributed to the economic downturn that occurred, the disease itself has had a much larger impact on the world.

Hindsight being what it is, medical experts now know that we should have implemented more effective public health measures at the outset of the virus spreading and with each successive wave. (See Chapters 3 and 4 for information about the pandemic and its effects on society.) Ending lockdowns earlier probably had economic benefits, but it resulted in higher COVID death rates — and with the knowledge the world gained from the 2020 pandemic, the global community can avoid making the same mistake twice.

All the people working to eliminate and eradicate diseases and viruses can't fully get rid of many of them after they take hold in a population. But that doesn't mean the world should give up trying.

Hundreds of Americans are still dying every day with COVID-19, and Long COVID affects millions of people. As global citizens, everyone needs to stay updated on the latest developments on COVID-19 (for example, from sources given in this chapter's introduction) and remain committed to health and hygiene practices that keep the virus at bay — including widespread isolation and lockdowns again, if governments and public health agencies deem them necessary.

You Can Catch COVID-19 from a Public Pool

SARS-CoV-2 is airborne and doesn't travel through water.

No evidence suggests that you can catch SARS-CoV-2 from public pools — or hot tubs, splash pads, or natural bodies of water such as lakes, rivers, ponds, and oceans. As long as the pool is properly disinfected with chlorine or bromine, don't worry about most other viruses or bacteria, either.

TIP

Like with any public space, use your best judgment about whether you consider it a healthy space to be in, and what steps you can take to maintain good hygiene. You may choose to mask at indoor water parks or in enclosed spaces, such as locker rooms.

All COVID-19 Treatments Are Created Equal

As of this writing, people have access to several different COVID-19 treatments, but not all treatments are right for everyone. *Each treatment has different degrees of efficacy, dosages, and impacts.*

I go over each current treatment in detail in Chapter 8, so check out that chapter if you need more information about specific medications and treatment plans. No one treatment is better than the others; how well they work depends on the particular patient and several factors, such as

>> **How severe the case of COVID-19 is:** Severe symptoms (such as difficulty breathing) may require more invasive treatments (possibly a ventilator) than do milder symptoms (such as body aches) which you can treat by taking an over-the-counter (OTC) pain killer.

>> **How long ago the patient became infected:** If it's been five or less days since you developed your first symptom, you may be able to start on certain medications that will shorten or lessen the impact of your illness.

>> **The patient's age and overall health status:** Seniors and people who have existing health conditions (such as heart or lung disease, diabetes, or obesity) may require more intensive treatment or treatment that lasts longer than people who aren't dealing with these factors.

>> **Whether the patient can tolerate IV or oral medication:** Some people get very nauseous or feel pain during IV treatments, so their doctor may prescribe pills. For those who can handle it without feeling too sick or painful, their doctor may opt to give them a COVID-19 treatment through an IV infusion.

Throughout the pandemic, we in the medical community also discovered which treatments didn't work. These ineffective treatments include hydroxychloroquine, ivermectin, IV vitamin C, plasma, and stem cells. Not only do these medications do nothing to treat COVID-19, but they also can have serious, and sometimes fatal, side effects.

If you want to seek treatment for COVID-19, make an appointment with your doctor to discuss what option is best for you.

WARNING

Don't take anyone else's medication — ever. Even if it worked for them, it won't necessarily work for you. And more importantly, taking medication that's not prescribed for you can cause extreme illness.

IN THIS CHAPTER

» **Expanding vaccine technology and telemedicine**

» **Acquiring new habits: Food delivery and masking**

» **Recognizing the need for mental healthcare**

» **Enjoying home, family, and new work attitudes**

» **Changing how you interact with the news**

Chapter **13**

Almost Ten Ways Life Changed after COVID-19

A lthough the 2020 COVID-19 pandemic happened years ago, people around the world still feel the effects. From scientific advances to people forming new habits (such as masking and utilizing food delivery services) that have become mainstream, life changed permanently in many ways.

Many people have found some changes challenging to get used to, while they welcome other changes. But one thing's for sure: Your life after the pandemic doesn't look like the one you had before it.

Vaccine Innovation

During the 2020 COVID-19 pandemic, researchers had to move fast to develop vaccines and other medical care to stop the SARS-CoV-2 virus from spreading so far and fast. And their efforts worked — scientists developed a COVID-19 vaccine in about 11 months. That's an amazing feat, as compared to the previous record of five years (that's 60 months) that scientists took to develop the mumps vaccine in 1967.

Working quickly and creatively to battle the outbreak made scientists more adept at using mRNA technology to develop and advance COVID-19 vaccines, but they can apply the same approach and technology beyond that specific treatment. (Check out Chapter 6 for more about the vaccines' technology.) Even though the 2020 pandemic is over, scientists still use what they discovered during its crisis to streamline clinical testing for other vaccines and medical innovations *without* compromising safety.

Increased Availability of Telemedicine

Because COVID-19 is so contagious, and hospitals and doctor's offices were short staffed and overrun during the pandemic, doctors relied on telemedicine like never before to provide healthcare services from afar. *Telemedicine* involves using telecommunications technology to allow patients to receive diagnosis and treatment from their healthcare team remotely — without going into a medical facility.

Pre-pandemic, researchers hadn't studied telemedicine in depth, and medical professionals didn't commonly use telemedicine technology. During the pandemic, physicians used the technology exponentially more, and researchers studied telemedicine's impact more thoroughly. According to the paper "The State of Telehealth Before and After the COVID-19 Pandemic," by Julia Shaver, M.D. (published in the December 2022 issue of *Primary Care: Clinics in Office Practice*), telemedicine visits in the U.S. during the first three months of the pandemic increased by 766 percent.

Doctors and researchers found that using telemedicine was safer and more efficient when treating patients who had COVID-19, especially in rural areas. Normally, rural medical facilities transfer their sickest patients to larger facilities for the proper care, but because COVID-19 had all hospitals everywhere at or beyond capacity with patients, rural facilities had to figure out how to meet patient needs on their own. Doctors started using telemedicine more to reach and care for these patients.

As of this writing, the number of physicians across the U.S. who are using telemedicine has doubled since 2020. Like with many things in medicine (and in life), using telemedicine has both pros and cons.

For the pros, telemedicine

>> Continues to offer patients fast and easy access to care and gives doctors across the globe access to patients, regardless of location

>> Reduces the burden on medical infrastructure and decreases exposure to infectious diseases by not requiring in-person office or hospital visits

>> Remains especially useful in psychiatric care and medical visits that don't require a physical examination, such as follow-up visits for high blood pressure, diabetes, or depression

For the cons, telemedicine

>> Doesn't allow for all aspects of patient examination. Although we doctors are figuring out how to direct patients to perform some physical evaluation themselves, doctors just can't do many parts of the physical examination (for example, listening to the heart and lungs, or properly examining the abdomen) remotely.

>> Requires online access, which can be a problem for some patients in rural areas, as well as in the inner cities.

Increased Use of Food Delivery Services

When lockdowns and stay-at-home orders happened during the pandemic, consumers significantly reduced their visits to or stopped going to restaurants and retail stores altogether. To keep revenue coming in and meet the needs of their customers, many food service and retail businesses increased their delivery services — or added them to their offerings for the first time.

Consumers used online companies such as Uber Eats and Amazon more heavily to get meals, groceries, and household supplies.

According to the September 2021 report by Edison Trends ("Global Food Delivery Trends 2018 vs 2021"), U.S. food delivery increased by 96 percent during the pandemic, and the trajectory has continued. In 2021, food delivery transactions increased by

>> 171 percent in the U.K.

>> 86 percent in Canada

>> 58 percent in the U.S.

>> 30 percent in Australia

After the pandemic ended and restaurants opened up again for dine-in service, some people returned to their pre-pandemic delivery usage levels, but for many people, the pandemic showed them how using food delivery apps saves them valuable time and effort, so it's a habit that's here to stay.

Masking in Public

Even before the COVID-19 pandemic in 2020, public masking was very common in large Asian cities, and in some Asian communities in the U.S. But general-public masking wasn't popular in the U.S. or other Western countries.

After the pandemic began, people around the world wore masks as a key strategy to stop spreading COVID-19, and masking became a mainstream habit for much of the global population. Even though masking became less vital when vaccines and treatments became available, masking has remained mainstream.

In the post-pandemic world, people often still wear masks in public. People have become more used to wearing them in crowded spaces, during cold and flu seasons, when traveling, or when they feel under the weather. Many people keep multiple masks in multiple places — their homes, cars, and offices — as a regular habit.

Impact on Mental Wellness

According to the 2022 COVID-19 Practitioner Impact Survey, published by the American Psychological Association in November 2022, six in ten psychologists say they don't have openings for new patients.

This high demand for therapy illustrates how people in the U.S. are still experiencing and trying to get treatment for their mental health issues. Although many Americans struggled with mental illness before the pandemic, the pandemic worsened many pre-existing mental illnesses because people were isolated from their support systems and didn't have acces to their in-person therapies. And although some people can get the treatment they need, many people are still suffering.

A majority of the psychologists surveyed by the American Psychological Association note a marked uptick in patients who are dealing with anxiety, depression, and trauma, and that the demand for services continues to remain high. Specifically, 51 percent of psychologists reported seeing higher rates of teens seeking therapy since the beginning of the pandemic. Causes include

>> Schools shutting down and moving to remote education, which contributed to feelings of isolation for many young adults

>> Fear that many teens felt while living through sickness and watching their loved ones get sick or even die — especially older, much beloved grandparents

In response, more schools are hiring social workers, psychologists, and other mental health professionals to tend to the needs of these students and families while they continue to recover from the pandemic — and seek ongoing treatment beyond COVID-19 counseling. Schools, parents, and students alike are prioritizing mental health and wellness in the post-pandemic world more than they did before the pandemic, which can not only benefit them individually, but also benefit society as a whole.

Un-Retiring and Not Retiring

During the pandemic, millions of U.S. workers retired early, but with supply chain issues and inflation increasing the cost of living, many people are coming out of retirement and re-entering the workforce. According to T. Rowe Price's April 2023 Retirement Saving & Spending Study, approximately 20 percent of retirees are back to working either full time or part time.

Additionally, according to the June 2022 Transamerica Retirement Survey, 40 percent of respondents have added three to five years, and 35 percent had added nearly a decade, to their expected work years. One of the reasons for this trend is that the average American nest egg fell by 11 percent in 2022 to $86,869, down from $98,800 in 2021. On top of that, Americans think they need approximately 20 percent more money than they originally planned for retirement.

Even for people who didn't retire early, the lost wages from reduction in hours or similar cutbacks during the pandemic have put them behind their financial goals, and researchers expect people to continue to work longer to make up for it.

Increased desire for being outdoors or at home — even though the 2020 pandemic is over — and the popularity of outdoor spaces and events continues. Many restaurants that added outdoor dining tables during the pandemic have kept them. According to the National Restaurant Association, 40 percent of consumers say they're more likely to choose a restaurant with outdoor seating.

Retail stores got creative with providing outdoor shopping spaces and special events to cater to customers who preferred to avoid indoor communal spaces during the pandemic, and many of those stores have continued to offer pop-up events, picnics, and other special events.

And at home, people have increased and improved their outdoor living spaces, getting creative with porches, yards, and even balconies. An April 2023 survey of 1,000 homeowners conducted by the Research Institute for Cooking and Kitchen Intelligence showed that 64 percent of survey responders have a greater desire to stay home now than before the pandemic, and more people are upgrading their homes with luxury spaces, such as kitchen wine or coffee stations.

The Great Resignation

The pandemic gave rise to an economic phenomenon called the Great Resignation, where many employees quit their jobs after re-evaluating their priorities and values.

For many people, experiencing serious illness or even deaths in the family as a result of COVID-19 caused them to feel that their nine-to-five jobs weren't as important as they thought they were pre-pandemic. Many employees

>> **Opted for family and fun:** Employees began to prefer spending time with family and engaging in activities that improve their quality and enjoyment of life over spending so much time working in an unfulfilling career.

Because of the move to remote schooling, where children had to stay home, remote working with the same or newfound employment became more popular. Workers thrived because they could spend more time with their family, cut down on commuting expenses, and conduct their work more efficiently and productively.

>> **Reassessed job features:** People left their jobs because they felt burnt out (especially in the healthcare sector), didn't receive strong enough benefits, and wanted more flexible scheduling. Remote working rose to the top of the list as the main feature employees sought out when they looked for new employment.

REMEMBER

These shifts in attitude and workplace seem to predict a permanent change. Many experts (such as Robert Sadow, the CEO and co-founder of Scoop Technologies, which puts out the Flex report — a collection of insights from more than 4,000 companies employing more than 100 million people globally) suggest that many workers will never return to the office at pre-pandemic levels and will never again settle for being unhappy at work, remote or not.

Explosion of News Consumption and Misinformation

Several factors have caused misinformation to spread in an explosive way during and after the pandemic. This misinformation is primarily, but not exclusively, related to medical care. During the pandemic, people spent much more time at home than they did beforehand, and during much of that at-home time, they used their computers and smartphones to consume the 24/7 news cycle.

Although staying updated on current news was helpful for people who wanted the latest information on COVID-19, mass media can also act as a source of inaccurate information — and good or bad, it spreads easily and quickly to people. During the pandemic, many people who didn't have much else to do consumed a lot of media, including misinformation that discouraged people from masking, getting appropriate treatment, and receiving the COVID-19 (and other) vaccines.

The pandemic has made it clear that people will always have to use caution when assessing the information that they get about COVID-19 (and any other news item, for that matter).

TIP

To ensure that you're getting accurate and factual information, cross-check the stories that you see or read. If a friend tells you about something that they heard, always make sure to check it out for yourself with a reputable source (or sources) — and that goes for news stories that you consume yourself! If you read a story about a COVID-19 update in one newspaper, see if you can find the same information in another source to confirm it. You can also check with the World Health Organization (WHO), the U.S. Centers for Disease Control and Prevention (CDC), and/or your local health department for the most accurate information.

Chapter **14**

Nine Ways to Prepare for the Next Pandemic

You can't talk about *if* the world will experience another global pandemic; you have to talk about *when* it will. During the 2020 COVID-19 pandemic, the global population experienced sickness, loss, and death on an astounding global scale. As of this writing, it remains one of the worst pandemics in U.S. and world history. And if history is any indicator, it won't be the last.

Using the COVID-19 pandemic as a teacher, in this chapter, I give nine suggestions for what the U.S. and other countries around the world can do now to prepare for the next pandemic so that it doesn't cause as much damage or death as COVID-19 did during the 2020 pandemic.

Modernize Data Tracking

Countries around the world, including the U.S., should take steps now to modernize their capacity to track national and local infectious disease statistics. As of this writing, many countries have the ability to leverage advanced technologies — such as artificial intelligence, big data analytics, and real-time surveillance systems — to benefit public health. Governments and public health agencies must better use this technology to detect emerging outbreaks, which then allows all countries and healthcare systems to execute timely interventions.

No country is an island when it comes to pandemics. When all countries have upgraded and interconnected disease-tracking systems, the data can give officials the early warnings that they need to keep their populations safe, allowing them to be proactive, rather than reactive, in the face of looming health crises. Consider these points for sharing the data-tracking wealth, so to speak:

>> **Setting everyone up:** Wealthier countries should help underserved countries procure the technology and infrastructure they need to monitor and react to healthcare needs.

>> **Organizing information:** Countries worldwide need to integrate and centralize their health databases now so that authorities across borders can collaborate and obtain a cohesive view of disease patterns, assess transmission rates, and pinpoint hotspots with heightened precision.

>> **Communicating between local and national levels:** In the U.S., local health departments need to better coordinate data on emerging infections with the Centers for Disease Control and Prevention (CDC).

Improve the PPE Supply Chain

Enhancing the global supply chain for personal protective equipment (PPE) is a critical step in preparing for future pandemics. During the 2020 COVID-19 pandemic, the sudden and huge jump in demand for PPE led to severe shortages, jeopardizing the safety of healthcare workers and the general public. Now, governments know they need to — and should — take steps to

>> Diversify the PPE manufacturing bases.

>> Stockpile strategic reserves.

>> Establish clear procurement protocols.

>> Invest in innovative and sustainable materials that can be used to make PPE.

A nimble and robust PPE supply chain not only keeps frontline responders safe, but also helps to instill public confidence.

Mass Testing

In the U.S. and in many other countries, local health departments must get faster at increasing their testing capability for emerging infectious disease threats. The departments can do so by providing funding for research and development, properly updating equipment and training, and devising easy-to-deploy public education campaigns.

When public health and government officials put a more robust testing infrastructure in place, they can more quickly and effectively conduct rapid identification, start isolation, and provide treatment to infected individuals. These measures help to slow down the transmission of a disease from the start. Conducting adequate testing

>> **Allows the medical community to get a clear picture** of a pandemic's trajectory early on and to promptly isolate cases and quarantine contacts.

>> **Helps government and agency officials make informed decisions** about resource allocation, containment measures, and public health strategies.

Maintain Preparations for Surges

To better handle the next pandemic, hospitals worldwide need to accurately calculate and equip themselves properly for their surge capacities. *Surge capacity* refers to a facility's ability to expand its operations to safely treat an abrupt and significant influx of patients.

To calculate surge capacity, officials typically evaluate the current number of available critical resources — such as ICU beds, ventilators, and medical staff — against the potential demand during a health crisis. They consider factors such as their local population's size, level of vulnerability, disease transmission rates, and past hospitalization rates.

Preparing for a surge now — when hospitals aren't in the midst of a pandemic — can help them ensure that they can provide immediate and effective care to patients and reduce the strain that they put on their overall healthcare system the next time a surge occurs.

The 2020 COVID-19 pandemic showed that many hospitals weren't prepared to handle their surges and had difficulty caring for everyone who needed care. As always, funding is a key factor. Advocating for proper funding for healthcare infrastructure now — before we need it again — is critical to ongoing preparedness, including

>> **Regularly maintaining equipment and properly training staff:** This preparation is the ethical responsibility of all healthcare providers.

>> **Ensuring that all patients have access to a healthcare facility:** In the U.S., *safety net hospitals* (those that primarily care for patients insured by the government) bore the brunt of the COVID-19 pandemic and have been traditionally underfunded and therefore unable to prepare for patient surges.

Fight Misinformation

When news agencies, public figures, and even private citizens on social media share misinformation about a public health crisis, they can spread fear, stigmatize sick individuals, and hinder the effective implementation of public health measures. On top of that, spreading false remedies or treatments can jeopardize public health and divert attention from effective interventions.

When the public is misinformed, they may distrust the efforts of healthcare agencies and resist appropriate safety guidelines, such as masking, vaccinations, social distancing, lockdowns, or other measures put into place to stop the disease from spreading.

To build trust and collaboration among the public that can hold fast during times of public health crises, governments and private companies should continue to combat misinformation by

- » **Supporting and collaborating with independent fact- checking organizations that quickly debunk false claims:** Social media sites and other public websites and apps can integrate these fact checks directly into their systems to notify users of disputed content.

- » **Committing to transparency:** Public and private leadership should provide regular, clear, and consistent updates about public health (and other crisis) situations. They must also maintain open channels of communication, such as press conferences, official websites, and public service announcements, to give the public access to reliable sources of information.

- » **Investing in media literacy campaigns:** These campaigns can show the public how to distinguish credible sources from unreliable ones. Developing these critical-thinking skills helps individuals become more resistant to false or misleading narratives.

Preserve Animal Habitats

Preserving animal habitats and protecting them from human encroachment is a crucial strategy in reducing the risk of future pandemics. When humans disturb or remove animal habitats, they increase the risk of people having direct interactions with wildlife — which, in turn, increases the opportunities for them to contract *zoonotic pathogens* (infections that are spread between people and animals). See Chapter 3 for more about zoonotic infections.

Governments and public lands agencies need to protect animal habitats from overdevelopment and human entry, and the general public needs to respect all rules and limits in place to protect wildlife. Additionally, preserving animal habitats helps reduce the likelihood of future pandemics by

- » **Maintaining ecological balance:** When humans disrupt animal habitats, they can unintentionally alter the natural order of species. For example, if humans destroy certain predatory animals that prey on animals that are more susceptible to infections or serve as reservoirs for certain diseases, those prey animals increase in population, which increases the risk for diseases to spread to humans.

>> **Protecting biodiversity:** Scientists haven't yet fully proven it, but they have a lot of evidence that suggests, in diverse ecosystems, many pathogens get diluted among a variety of species, some of which aren't biologically capable of transmitting certain diseases, so the virus ends there instead of spreading. This dispersal is called the *dilution effect*.

>> **Decreasing stress-induced diseases:** Habitat destruction can stress wildlife populations, weakening their immune systems, which can allow pathogens to multiply unchecked.

Eliminate Live Animal Markets

To help reduce the chance of another global pandemic, public officials across the world need to eliminate live-animal markets. In addition, people and industries that raise animals for food need to keep those animals separate from other animal species, and regulations need to enforce that the facilities that raise those animals can't be placed in human population centers.

Currently, in live-animal markets, proprietors keep a variety of wild and domestic animals in close proximity, often under unsanitary conditions, which creates an environment that can easily lead to *spillover events,* where viruses move from one species of animal to another — and those viruses can turn into new viruses in the process. Many of these markets are in densely populated large cities, which increases the risk that zoonotic viruses encounter humans.

I talk more about these risks in Chapter 3, so turn there if you want details about the science of spillover events and how scientists believe that the 2020 COVID-19 pandemic most likely started with one.

Similarly, factory farms and other facilities that house vast numbers of animals densely packed together can also increase the risk for mutations and more virulent strains. Governments must reform and regulate these industries and practices by making changes such as

>> **Improving sanitary practices,** including regular and deep cleaning and disinfection, to prevent the introduction and spread of pathogens within farms.

>> **Reducing the number of animals per unit area** to lower stress, decrease disease transmission rates, and improve overall animal welfare.

>> **Ensuring that qualified veterinarians routinely inspect farms** and provide guidance on best practices to prevent disease outbreaks.

>> **Reducing antibiotic use** because overusing antibiotics can lead to antibiotic-resistant bacteria, which pose significant health risks. Officials need to promote prudent use of antibiotics and implement stricter regulations to eliminate non-therapeutic use.

Farmers frequently use antibiotics not only to treat sick animals, but also as *growth promoters,* which means that they add antibiotics to the feed of healthy animals to increase the weight of the animals and thus bring a higher price when they're sold or slaughtered.

Improve Overall Health Worldwide

The healthier the world's population is, the more likely people are to overcome illness and reduce the impact of another pandemic. Unfortunately, underdeveloped countries face limited healthcare infrastructure, lack of trained healthcare professionals, and inadequate access to medicines and vaccines. And even in developed countries, some marginalized populations lack ready access to the healthcare facilities and treatments that are available.

Wealthier nations and international organizations should support these underserved countries by investing and supporting their efforts to

>> **Promote overall wellness, nutrition, and preventative care** through public health campaigns and initiatives that teach citizens about how regular health check-ups are vital for healthy living, for example.

- >> **Improve treatment of chronic medical conditions,** such as hypertension, diabetes, and obesity. These treatments are much less expensive in the long run than treating the complications of these conditions, such as heart attacks, strokes, and amputated limbs.

- >> **Make medical services, such as community clinics and vaccination programs, free to the public** when the population can't afford them. Keeping people updated on their vaccines and healthy overall makes them less susceptible to infectious diseases because their bodies are more able to fight off germs.

Many other factors, beyond medical care, also help keep a population healthy, such as

- >> **Regular public sanitation services that include trash pickup:** Without trash management, waste breeds bacteria that can make people sick.

- >> **Access to clean water:** Dirty water can contain contaminants that make people extremely sick.

- >> **Proper housing:** When people live too close together, and without proper shelter, they can more easily and quickly transmit diseases.

- >> **Introducing hand hygiene and responsible antibiotic use as early as possible:** For example, introduce these ideas in schools so that people grow up knowing simple and effective steps to take to stop spreading germs.

Ensure Funding

In order to pay for all of the ideas and suggestions that I discuss in this chapter, governments, public health agencies, and medical providers need ongoing funding. Without proper funding, even the most advanced nations can get overwhelmed, leading to loss of life and socioeconomic instability.

Two good examples of successful funding efforts are the Global Fund to Fight AIDS, Tuberculosis and Malaria; and Gavi, the Vaccine

Alliance. Although they primarily focus on specific diseases, their frameworks — centered on global collaboration, resource pooling, and healthcare capacity building — serve as exemplary models. Additionally, the Global Health Security Agenda (GHSA) aims to help countries build capacity to prevent, detect, and respond to infectious disease threats. U.S.-based funding initiatives include

» **The Public Health Emergency Preparedness (PHEP) cooperative agreement:** Led by the Centers for Disease Control and Prevention (CDC), this agreement provides critical funding to states to bolster their abilities to respond to various public health threats, including infectious diseases, natural disasters, and biological, chemical, nuclear, and radiological events.

» **Hospital Preparedness Program (HPP):** Administered by the Office of the Assistant Secretary for Preparedness and Response (ASPR), this program provides funding to healthcare systems to increase their preparedness for public health emergencies.

» **The Emerging Pandemic Threats (EPT) program:** Run by the U.S. Agency for International Development (USAID), this program focuses on detecting and responding to viruses that have pandemic potential, especially in regions where human-animal interactions are frequent and pose a high risk of disease emergence.

» **Biomedical Advanced Research and Development Authority (BARDA) investments:** BARDA consistently invests in the advanced research and development of medical countermeasures, such as vaccines, therapeutics, and diagnostics, specifically for threats that include pandemic influenza and other emerging infectious diseases.

Investment in, and expansion of, such programs ensures that when the next pandemic strikes, the world doesn't have to scramble for resources, but is poised with well-funded, established mechanisms to respond promptly and effectively.

Index

Numerics

3D printing technology, 60

A

Agency for Healthcare Research and Quality (AHRQ), 164

AI (artificial intelligence), 60

airborne transmission, 75–76

Americans with Disabilities Act (ADA), 155–156

anaphylaxis, 90

animal habitats, preserving, 205–206

antibodies, 27

antibody tests, 106

antivirals
Lagevrio, 124–125
overview, 120–121
Paxlovid, 122–123
Veklury, 121–122

arthralgia, 150–151

artificial intelligence (AI), 60

assisted-living communities, 58–59

at-home tests, 107–108

autoantibodies, 137

automation, 61

automotive industry, 69

azithromycin, 127

B

BARDA (Biomedical Advanced Research and Development Authority) investments, 209

benzocaine, 128

Bill and Melinda Gates Foundation, 162

Biomedical Advanced Research and Development Authority (BARDA) investments, 209

bivalent vaccines, 86

Black, indigenous, and people of color (BIPOC) populations, 138

boosters, 29, 92–93

Brookings Metro, 161

burnout
healthcare workers, 66–67
teachers, 64–65

C

cardiac decline, 145–146

cardiac stress test, 146

CARES (Coronavirus Aid, Relief, and Economic Security) Act of 2020, 54

Centers for Disease Control and Prevention (CDC)
Public Health Emergency Preparedness cooperative agreement, 209
recommendations for mRNA vaccine, 91–92
role in response to pandemic, 42–43

CEPI (Coalition for Epidemic Preparedness Innovations), 41

Cheat Sheet for book, 3

China National Accreditation Service for Conformity Assessment (CNAS), 36

chronic COVID. See Long COVID

close contact, 114

cloth masks, 95–97

S

About the Author

Edward K. Chapnick, M.D., holds several positions at Maimonides Medical Center in Brooklyn, New York, including Director of the Division of Infectious Diseases, Executive Vice Chair of the Department of Medicine, and Hospital Epidemiologist. His practice in the specialty of infectious diseases and travel medicine includes the treatment of patients who have a wide range of problems, such as HIV, antibiotic-resistant bacterial infections, and of course, COVID-19.

Dr. Chapnick received his medical degree from the State University of New York (SUNY) Downstate Medical Center and completed his training in Internal Medicine and Infectious Diseases at Maimonides Medical Center. He's a fellow of the American College of Physicians, the Infectious Diseases Society of America, and the Society for Healthcare Epidemiology of America. His activities also include teaching, and he's a professor of clinical medicine at the SUNY Downstate Health Sciences University in Brooklyn. Dr. Chapnick has numerous publications in peer-reviewed medical literature and is actively engaged in clinical research.

Dedication

This book is dedicated to Stephan L. Kamholz, M.D., who was Chair of the Department of Medicine at Maimonides Medical Center until he died from COVID-19 in June 2020. My friend, colleague, mentor, and boss, Steve was the epitome of a physician-educator. Despite our pleas not to do so, he insisted on coming to work every day during the pandemic as our leader. I pay tribute to Steve and to all healthcare workers and first responders who perished during the pandemic.

Author's Acknowledgments

I want to thank the team at John Wiley & Sons, Inc. for providing me with the opportunity to participate in this important project. The core team that I worked with to bring this book to fruition includes Sarah Sypniewski, contributor; Tracy Boggier, Senior Acquisitions Editor; Leah Michael, Project Editor; and Laura K. Miller, Copy Editor. You've helped through every step in the process of planning and writing the book, and you've been patient with my incomplete knowledge of the editorial and formatting process. Sarah, it has once again been a great pleasure to work with you and learn from you. It was truly an honor to work with such a capable and professional team.

Publisher's Acknowledgments

Senior Acquisitions Editor:
Tracy Boggier

Contributor: Sarah Sypniewski

Development Editor: Leah Michael

Copy Editor: Laura K. Miller

Proofreader: Debbye Butler

Production Editor:
Tamilmani Varadharaj

Cover Image: © wildpixel/iStock/
Getty Images

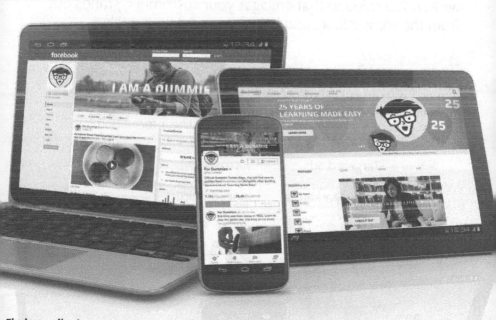

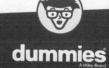

Leverage the power

Dummies is the global leader in the reference category and one of the most trusted and highly regarded brands in the world. No longer just focused on books, customers now have access to the dummies content they need in the format they want. Together we'll craft a solution that engages your customers, stands out from the competition, and helps you meet your goals.

Advertising & Sponsorships

Connect with an engaged audience on a powerful multimedia site, and position your message alongside expert how-to content. Dummies.com is a one-stop shop for free, online information and know-how curated by a team of experts.

- Targeted ads
- Video
- Email Marketing
- Microsites
- Sweepstakes sponsorship

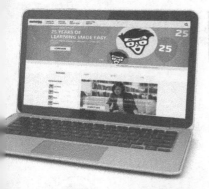

20 **MILLION**
PAGE VIEWS
EVERY SINGLE MONTH

15
MILLION
UNIQUE
VISITORS PER MONTH

43%
OF ALL VISITORS
ACCESS THE SITE
VIA THEIR MOBILE DEVICES

700,000 NEWSLETTER
SUBSCRIPTION
TO THE INBOXES OF
300,000 UNIQUE INDIVIDUALS
EVERY WEEK

# of dummies

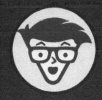

Custom Publishing

Reach a global audience in any language by creating a solution that will differentiate you from competitors, amplify your message, and encourage customers to make a buying decision.

- Apps
- Books
- eBooks
- Video
- Audio
- Webinars

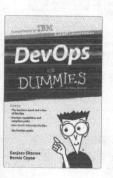
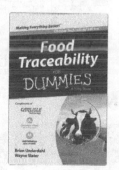
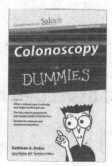
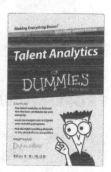

Brand Licensing & Content

Leverage the strength of the world's most popular reference brand to reach new audiences and channels of distribution.

For more information, visit dummies.com/biz

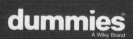

PERSONAL ENRICHMENT

Staying Sharp	Facebook	Guitar	Investing	Beekeeping	Digital Photography
9781119187790	9781119179030	9781119293354	9781119293347	9781119310068	9781119235606
USA $26.00	USA $21.99	USA $24.99	USA $22.99	USA $22.99	USA $24.99
CAN $31.99	CAN $25.99	CAN $29.99	CAN $27.99	CAN $27.99	CAN $29.99
UK £19.99	UK £16.99	UK £17.99	UK £16.99	UK £16.99	UK £17.99

Meditation	Pregnancy	Samsung Galaxy S7	iPhone	Crocheting	Nutrition
9781119251163	9781119235491	9781119279952	9781119283133	9781119287117	9781119130246
USA $24.99	USA $26.99	USA $24.99	USA $24.99	USA $24.99	USA $22.99
CAN $29.99	CAN $31.99	CAN $29.99	CAN $29.99	CAN $29.99	CAN $27.99
UK £17.99	UK £19.99	UK £17.99	UK £17.99	UK £16.99	UK £16.99

PROFESSIONAL DEVELOPMENT

Windows 10	AutoCAD	Excel 2016	QuickBooks 2017	macOS Sierra	LinkedIn	Windows 10
9781119311041	9781119255796	9781119293439	9781119281467	9781119280651	9781119251132	9781119310563
USA $24.99	USA $39.99	USA $26.99	USA $26.99	USA $29.99	USA $24.99	USA $34.00
CAN $29.99	CAN $47.99	CAN $31.99	CAN $31.99	CAN $35.99	CAN $29.99	CAN $41.99
UK £17.99	UK £27.99	UK £19.99	UK £19.99	UK £21.99	UK £17.99	UK £24.99

SharePoint 2016	Fundamental Analysis	Networking	Office 2016	Office 365	Salesforce.com	Coding
9781119181705	9781119263593	9781119257769	9781119293477	9781119265313	9781119239314	9781119293323
USA $29.99	USA $26.99	USA $29.99	USA $26.99	USA $24.99	USA $29.99	USA $29.99
CAN $35.99	CAN $31.99	CAN $35.99	CAN $31.99	CAN $29.99	CAN $35.99	CAN $35.99
UK £21.99	UK £19.99	UK £21.99	UK £19.99	UK £17.99	UK £21.99	UK £21.99